Contribution of Rational Drug Design for Efficacious Target Interactions

Humeera rafeeq

Afiya ansari

Ms. Tasleem

ISBN:1535419032
ISBN-13:9781535419031

Contents

PREFACE

As chemistry is a wide subject with its scope at peak, and is further emerging. I feel great pleasure in enlightening and presenting the informative text on 'Contribution of Rational Drug Design for Efficacious Drug Interactions'. The book aims mainly at the role and importance of Rational Drug Design making the compound able to bring its best in terms of stability, interactions and increasing its pharmaceutical activity. The complexity of the matter is minimized aiding the readers with the ease of understanding.

1 RATIONAL DRUG DESIGN

1.1- Introduction

In the discovering of lead compound many methods were used. Once the lead compound was discovered, it is used in drug designing as the starting point (Fig 1.1). Drug designing focuses on various aims. An ultimate drug should be easily synthesized possessing high level of target activity, chemical stability, minimum side effects and good penetration property. Mainly it should be non toxic and posses satisfactory pharmacokinetic properties. In this chapter improved optimization in drug-target interactions can be done using various design strategies i.e. improving pharmacokinetic properties of the drugs. Design strategies which improve the interaction by increasing the ability of the drug to reach its desired site of action, with increased lifetime are mainly focused. The ability of the drug to reach its site of action is one of the most important pharmacokinetic properties. For e.g. If we consider a drug which have a high interacting property with its target site but is low in reaching its sight of action is basically a poor drug in its pharmacokinetic sense . The property of the drug to reach its site of action is also an important factor. Therefore, pharmacodynamics and pharmacokinetics of a drug should be equally balanced and have equal concern in deciding which strategies must be used.

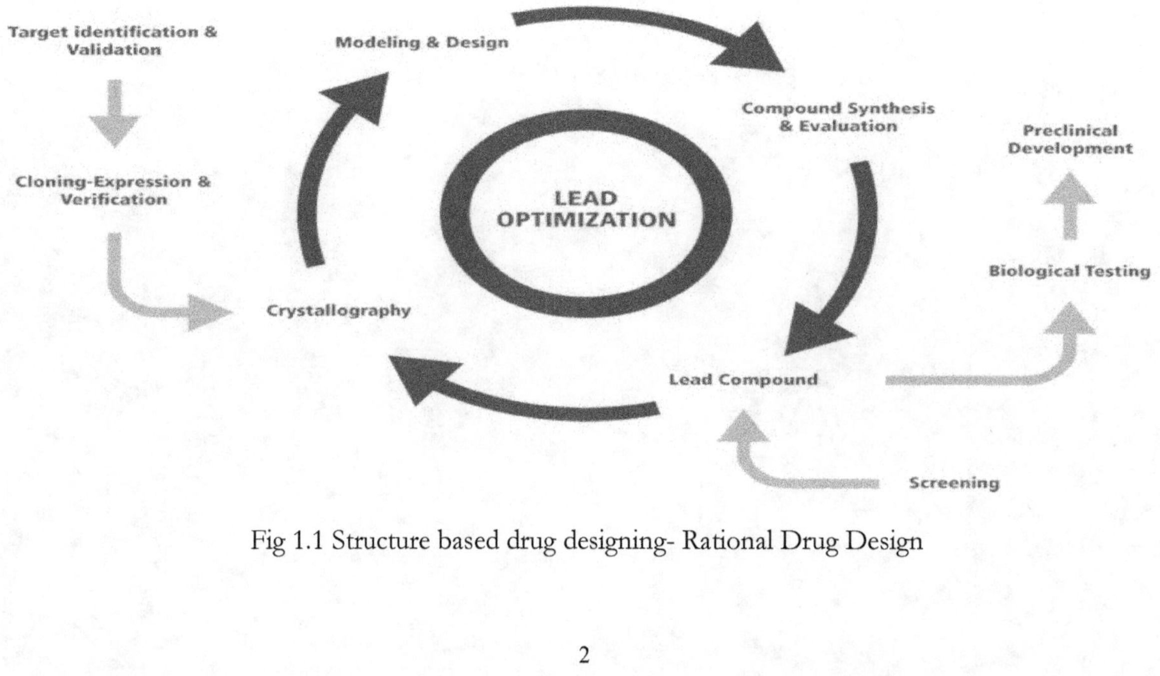

Fig 1.1 Structure based drug designing- Rational Drug Design

1.2- Structure-Activity Relationships (SAR)

Structure activity relationship mainly aims at discovering molecule parts which are important for its biological activity. After the discovery of lead compound which acts as a starting point, further its structure activity relationship is studied. If the drug bound with the targeted binding site is able to crystallize, its structure complex can be observed by the X-ray crystallography and further studied by the molecular modeling software. As the crystallization of the target structure or identification of target structure cannot be done, the X-ray crystallography and molecular modeling software may not be possible. In such cases, it is necessary to revert by synthesizing selected compounds in traditional method, which may slightly vary from original structure and studying which effect is seen on its biological activity. Various functional groups such as alkyl groups been present within the structure can assist either in the protected transport of the drug in the body to the site of action or helpful in binding to the targeted site. So, the functional groups present in a molecule and intermolecular bonds are recognized for better understanding drug target interactions. For example consider in case of morphine shown in Fig. 1.2

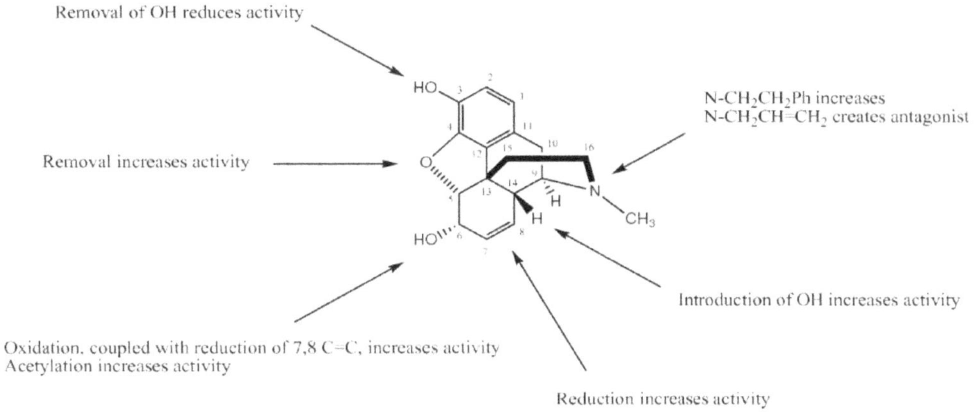

Fig 1.2 Morphine structure- indicating the effect of different functional groups on its biological activity

The recognizing of the functional groups in a particular molecule is important. A molecule may possess a biologically important part and other parts which possess no such actions. So, the original molecule is been taken and their analogue are been prepared by removing specific functional group. This analogue is been tested and compared to the compound, if the biological activity is been decreased then the functional group which has been removed possess an important role in drug action. In this manner, various analogues of the compounds are prepared and the tests are carried out indicating the effect of removal of specific functional groups, in these manner important functional groups required for its biological action can be easily identified. The recognizing task can be easily done based on how the necessary analogues are been synthesized. In case of lead, some analogues can be directly obtained by modification in the original molecule, while other analogues are best in total synthesis.

1.3 Binding Interactions

Role of Different Functional Groups in Binding

For different functional groups and their analogues various binding interactions are possible for its synthesis, to indicate whether these groups are helpful in binding or not. The role of functional groups in binding of the drug with the targeted site is discussed in detail in the below sections.

1.3.1- Aromatic ring

Hydrophobic interactions and van der Waals are commonly involved interactions with the binding site containing flat hydrophobic regions as they are planar and hydrophobic in nature. Any other analogues in which the ring gets less flatten as in the case of cyclohexane, the poor interaction between the molecule and the hydrophobic region can be seen (Fig 1.3.a). Cyclohexane when compared to an aromatic ring is bulky in its structure and is not capable to fit into the hydrophobic region of the binding site unlike aromatic ring which fits in perfectly due to the narrow slot rather its planar surface.

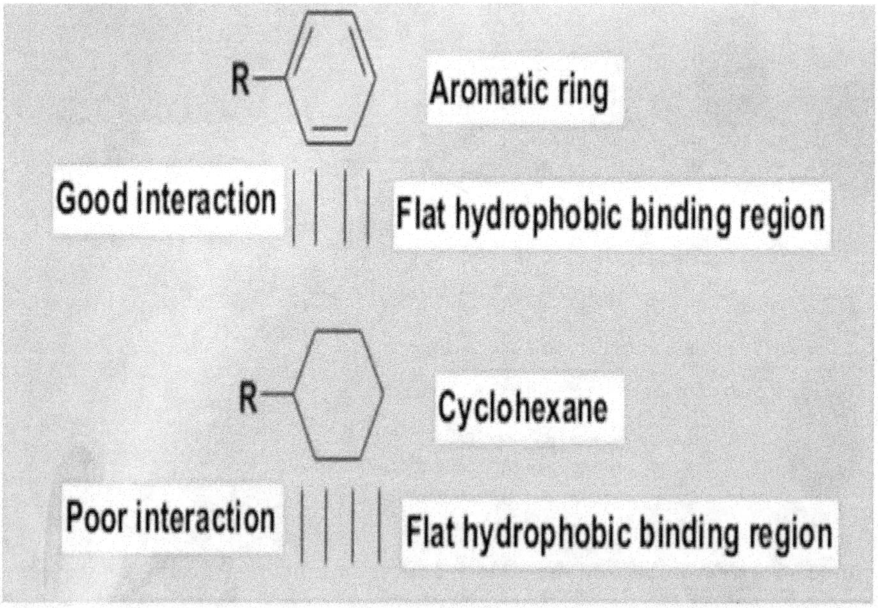

Fig 1.3.a comparison of aromatic ring and cyclohexane interactions

The amino acids such as Phenylalanine, tyrosine and tryptophan (Fig1.3.b) are highly hydrophobic due to hydrophobic nature of aromatic rings.

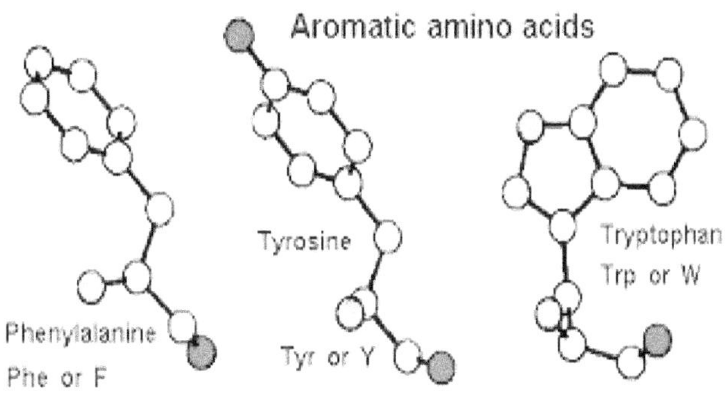

Fig 1.3.b Phenylalanine, tyrosine and tryptophan- the aromatic rings are highly hydrophobic

For most of the lead compounds, the aromatic rings cannot be easily converted into cyclohexane rings, and such analogues can be prepared normally by full synthesis method. By means of hydrogen bonding or induced dipole interactions, the interacting of aromatic rings with an ammonium ion is possible. For cyclohexyl analogue these interactions are not possible.

1.3.2- Ketones and Aldehydes

Many of the studied medicinal chemistry structures the ketone group is a common one. The carboxyl oxygen present in the planar group facilitates the hydrogen bonding with the binding site by acting as a hydrogen bond acceptor. Because of the presence of two lone pairs of electrons, two such hydrogen bonding interactions are possible at the carbonyl oxygen. These lone pairs are in the same plane as that of functional group as they are sp2 hybridized (Fig 1.3.c).

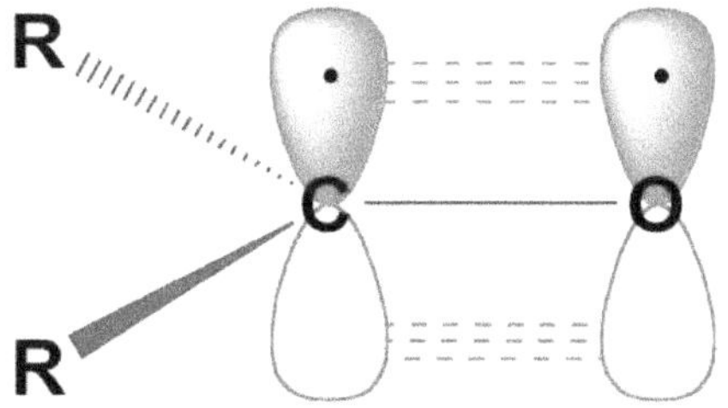

Fig 1.3.c hydrogen bonding at the carbonyl oxygen (sp2 hybridized- lone pairs at same plane)

The carbonyl oxygen of the ketone group also shows significant dipole moment making the dipole-dipole interaction possible at the binding site. In a lead compound it is possible to reduce a ketone group into an alcohol group by direct reaction. Tetrahedral geometry of an alcohol group from a planar one can be obtained due to changes in geometry of the functional group. Due to changes in the geometry, the magnitude and the orientation are altered for the dipole moment leading to the weakening of the existing hydrogen bond as well as dipole-dipole interactions. Many reactions are available which removes the oxygen completely by reducing a ketone group into an alkane one, but in the case of lead compounds these reactions are unpractical in medicinal chemistry studies. Due to high susceptibility of oxidation to carboxylic acids, aldehydes are the uncommon group in the drugs. However, they possess same reactivity as such of ketones and studying of similar analogues is possible (Fig 1.3.d).

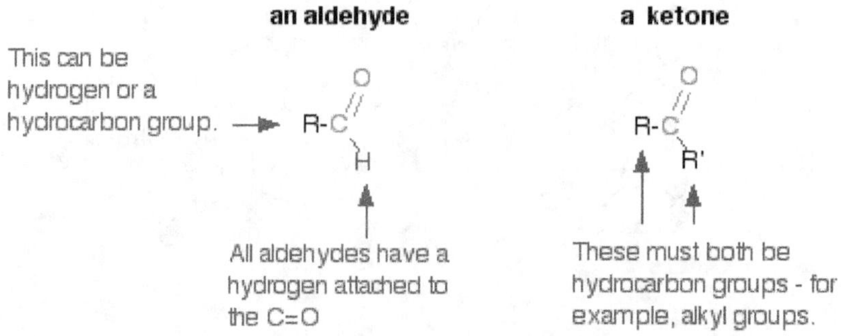

Fig 1.3.d showing oxidation in an aldehyde and a ketone group

1.3.3- Alcohols and Phenols

Many drugs contain alcohols and phenols as their functional groups which are generally involved in hydrogen bonding interactions. The hydrogen atom of the OH group acts as a hydrogen bond donor, whereas oxygen atom acts as acceptor of hydrogen bond. The hydrogen bond is indicated with an arrow mark. One or all the possible interactions may play an essential role in the binding of the drug to its binding site. Synthesis of methyl ether or ester analogue will be applicable in testing this, because they are possible chances of disruption of bonding in either analogue. Consider methyl ether as shown in the Fig 1.3.e. The hydroxyl group contains a proton which is involved in hydrogen bonding as it acts as hydrogen bond donor, and if the proton is removed it leads to the loss of hydrogen bond. This is one of the two reasons because of which the ether might prevent the formation of hydrogen bond. The second reason is that due to the removal of proton, the oxygen atom present in the molecule may act as hydrogen bond acceptor but not to the same extend as to that of an original compound because the increase in the methyl group may obstruct the close approach to that of a previous one and disrupts the hydrogen bonding.

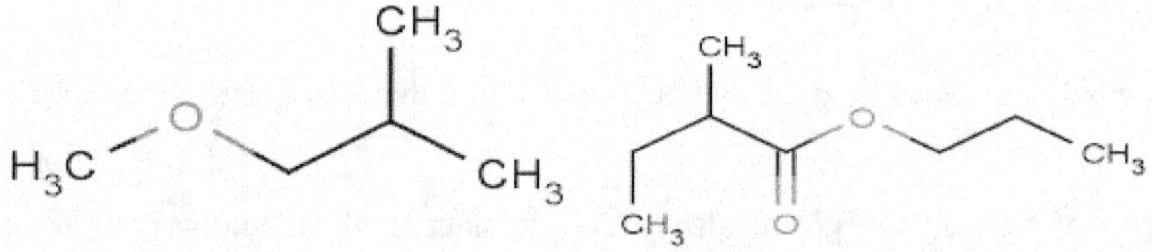

Fig 1.3.e methyl ether and ester showing possible hydrogen bonding interactions for functional groups (alcohol and phenol)

Complete disruption or prevention of hydrogen bond is not done but the bond may be weakened when compared to that of original molecule. The same case can be seen with that of an ester analogue that is, it cannot act as hydrogen bond donor but still there is a possibility of ester analogue to act as hydrogen bond acceptor, but the increased acyl group than that the methyl group disrupts the hydrogen bonding interactions as that of original one. Difference can be seen in the electronic properties of an alcohol and an ester. A resonance structure is formed due to the weak pull on electrons by the carboxyl group from the adjacent oxygen. This interaction will be less effective than the hydrogen bond acceptor as lone pair of electrons is involved. The carbonyl oxygen present in the molecule may act as hydrogen bond acceptor, but the carbonyl group is relatively in different positive in the molecule and is not able to form such interaction as that of hydrogen bond present at the binding site in original molecule. Alcohols and phenols can be easily acetylated to esters such as in case of morphine. Ethers and esters can be formed from both alcohols and phenols to observe the effect on binding. OH interacting with the binding site is been seen, but aromatic ring can also take part in interactions at intermolecular levels.

1.3.4- Alkenes

Alkenes are hydrophobic and planar like that of aromatic rings. Alkenes can interact by interacting with the hydrophobic regions with the binding site by means of van der Waals hydrophobic interactions (Fig 1.3.f).

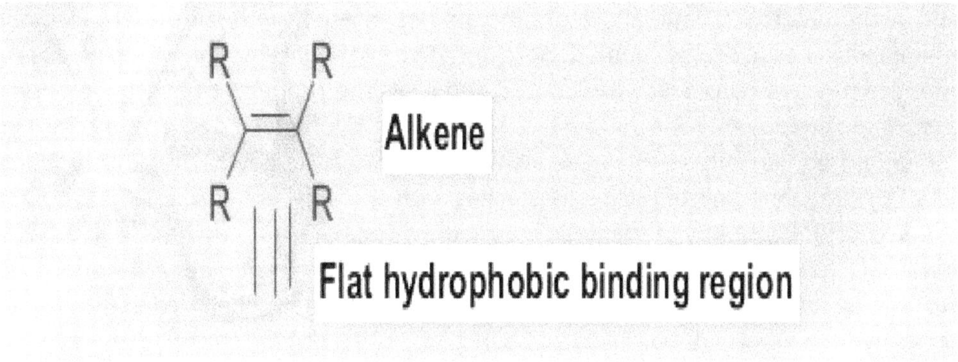

Fig 1.3.f hydrophobic interactions in alkenes

The activity of saturated analogue which is equivalent to original molecule is worth testing, because the alkyl region which is saturated is in excess and is unable to approach the adjacent binding site region so closely. Alkenes can be reduced easily than the aromatic rings; therefore it is possible to synthesize the saturated analogue from lead compound directly.

1.3.5- Amines

Many drugs in medicinal chemistry contain amines as a functional group and it is an extremely important one. Their interactions involve hydrogen bond donor and hydrogen bond acceptor facilitating hydrogen bonding. One lone pair of electron is present in the nitrogen atom of amine group and interacts by hydrogen bonding by acting as hydrogen bond acceptor (Fig 1.3.g).

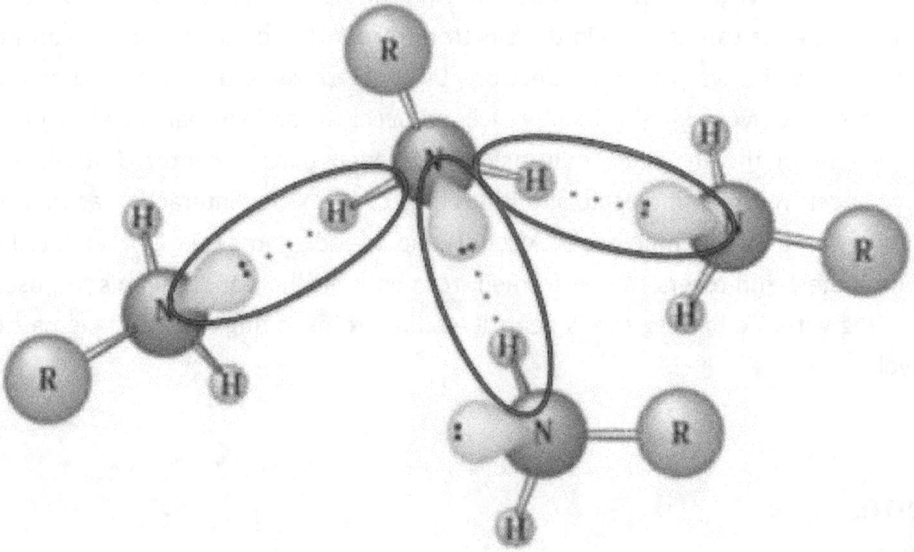

Fig 1.3.g Presence of lone pair of electrons in nitrogen atom (hydrogen bonding between amines)

N-H groups are present in primary (10) and secondary (20) amines and they act as hydrogen bond donors. As the lone pair present in the heteroaromatic and aromatic amines interact with the heteroaromatic and aromatic ring, so these amine can act as hydrogen bond donors only. When the interaction of amine at target binding site occurs, the amines are protonated i.e. they are ionized and loses the property of hydrogen bond acceptor. But it can still form a stronger hydrogen bond because it still acts as hydrogen bond donor; the hydrogen bond is stronger than of unionized. An amide analogue can be studied to test whether interactions are hydrogen bonding or ionic. In this the lone pair of nitrogen attaches with the adjacent carbonyl group preventing it to act as hydrogen bond acceptor. Possibility of the ionic interactions to take place can be observed as the protonation is prevented. Primary (1^0) and secondary amines (2^0) can relatively form secondary (2^0) and tertiary (3^0) amines respectively, and this direct reactions are possible for lead compounds. The secondary (2^0) amide formed is obstructed to act as hydrogen bond donor inspite of N-H group present, due to the excess of acyl group present. Amides cannot be formed directly from the tertiary (3^0) amines, but if a methyl group is present as an alkyl group it can be easily removed using vinyloxycarbonyl chloride (VOC-Cl) in the formation of secondary (2^0) amide which later can be converted to amide. Positive effects have been seen in morphine analogues synthesis by this demethylation reaction (Fig 1.3.h) and this reaction is an extremely used reaction.

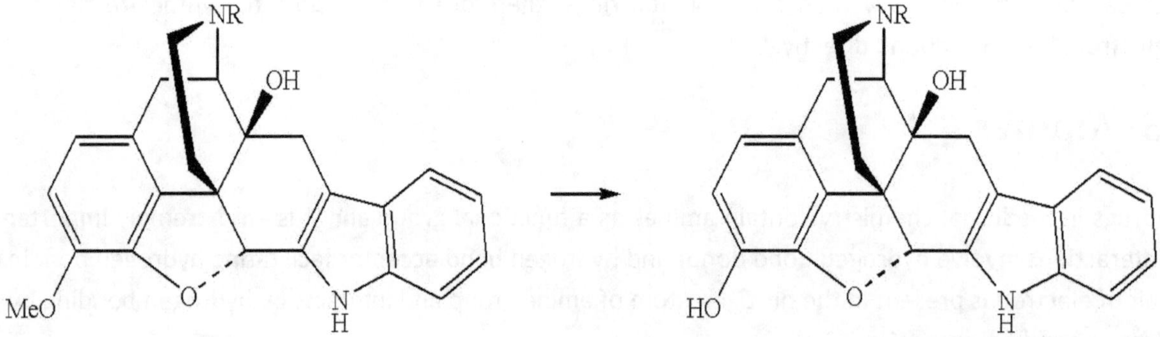

(1) R = Me
Oxymorphindole-3-methyl ether

Oxymorphindole

Fig 1.3h demethylation of morphine analogues

1.3.6- Amides

Peptides and polypeptides are the commonly studied lead compounds in medicinal chemistry, consists of amino acids which are linked by amide or peptide bonds. Amides with the binding sites are likely to interact by hydrogen bonding. The carbonyl oxygen has the ability to form 2 hydrogen bonds as it behaves as a hydrogen bond acceptor. The lone pairs are similar to that of amide group as they are in the same plane as sp2 hybridized orbitals. The nitrogen as it interacts with the adjacent carbonyl group is unable to behave as a hydrogen bond acceptor. N-H group is present in primary (1^0) and secondary (2^0) amides, allowing the possibility to act as hydrogen bond donor. Secondary amide is the most common amide among the peptide lead compounds. Certain analogues can be prepared for the testing of possible binding interactions (Fig 1.3.i)

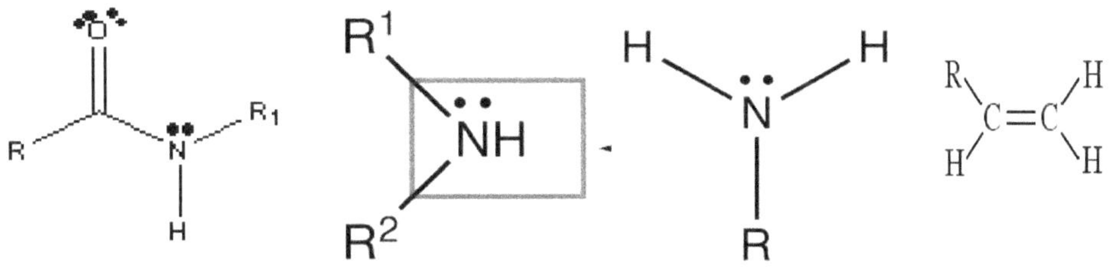

Fig 1.3.i Secondary amide secondary amine primary amine alkene

Except the amines (10, 20) almost all the analogues can be used to identify whether amide group acts as hydrogen bond donor, to identify whether amide acts as hydrogen bond acceptor amines and alkenes can be tested. Due to the partial double bond the amide group does not rotate and is planar. At equivalent position secondary amine, tertiary amine and ketone analogues poses single bond which can rotate. Due to this the relative positions of amide group on either side of binding groups is altered leading to binding loss even if amide group itself is uninvolved in binding. Hence, activity loss does not definitely mean that amide group is essential as binding group. With the above groups, it is right to say that NH2 group is not is important if the activity is preserved. Similarly no activity can be found by carboxylic acid and primary amine, mainly due to loss of essential binding groups at one half of molecule. These specific analogues can only be worth for taking in consideration if the peripheral part of molecule contains amide group. Alkenes acts as a useful test analogue as it cannot rotate i.e. planar and can neither act as hydrogen bond acceptor nor hydrogen bond donor. Hence the above described analogues should be prepared by means of full synthesis several analogues of amide can be attained directly from the lead compound as amides are stable functional groups in relation to other groups.

1.3.7- Thiols and Ethers

The (S-H) thiol group acts as a good ligand in relation to zinc ion and is thus incorporated into many drugs which are designed for inhibiting enzymes which contain zinc cofactor. These enzymes are called as zinc metallo proteinases. If the thiol group is present in lead compound, the relative alcohol can be tested. This leads to weak interactions with transition metal like zinc.An ether group (ROR) acts as hydrogen bond acceptor between oxygen atoms. The test can be carried out by on neighboring alkyl group by increasing the size to see if it reduces the capability of group to participate in hydrogen bonding. Significant decrease in binding affinity is seen in analogues where oxygen is used in place methylene (CH2) isostere.

1.3.8- Alkyl Groups and Carbon Skeleton

The carbon skeleton and alkyl substituent's of lead compound is hydrophobic in nature and binds to hydrophobic regions through hydrophobic interactions and Vander Waals forces to the binding site. The relation between alkyl substituent and binding site can be known by the synthesis of analogue lacking the substituent. These analogues if attached with carbon skeleton of molecule should generally be synthesized by full synthesis. If oxygen or nitrogen are present attached with the alkyl group it can be possible to detach the alkyl group from lead compound (for eg. demethylation of methyl ether using hydrogen bromide HBr Fig 1.3.j). Thus the activity of analogue is expected to get reduced if alkyl group undergone important hydrophobic interactions.

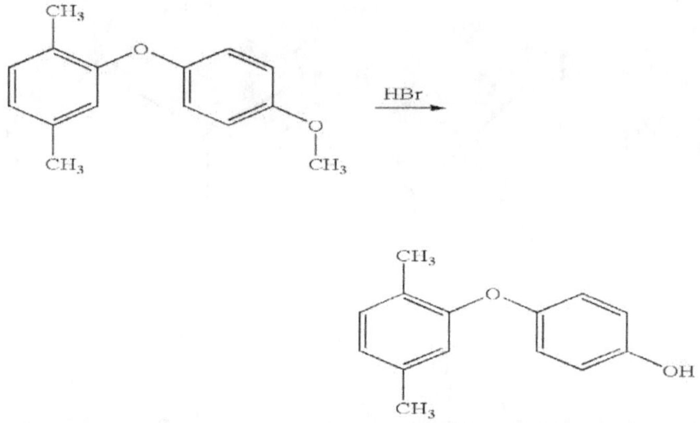

Fig 1.3.j demethylation of methyl ether using HBr

1.3.9- Other Functional Groups

Lead compounds may possess other functional groups in vast variety which shows no direct binding, but is important in other aspects. Functional groups such as nitro groups or nitriles have influenced on electronic properties of molecules. Whereas alkynes restrict the conformation or shape of molecule and functional groups such as aryl halides acts as metabolic blockers.

1.3.10- Quaternary Ammonium Salts

Quaternary ammonium salts interacts by ionic interactions with the carboxylate groups as they are ionized it can also interact between aromatic ring in binding site and quaternary ammonium ion by induced dipole interaction. The electron availability in the aromatic ring is decreased by the positively charged nitrogen atom thereby inducing dipole effect. The slightly positive edges, slightly negative ring face is observed in such a ring leading to possibility of interaction between quaternary ammonium positive ion and slightly negative aromatic ring faces. An analogue is been synthesized possessing a tertiary amine group replacing quaternary ammonium group exhibiting the necessity of these interactions. There is a possibility of a group to get ionized by protonation; this can be prevented by converting an amine group to amide. Acetylcholine a common neurotransmitter possessing quaternary ammonium group is assumed to bind with its target receptor at the binding site by means of induced dipole interactions and/or by ionic bonding exhibited by change in the ion channel (Fig 1.3.k).

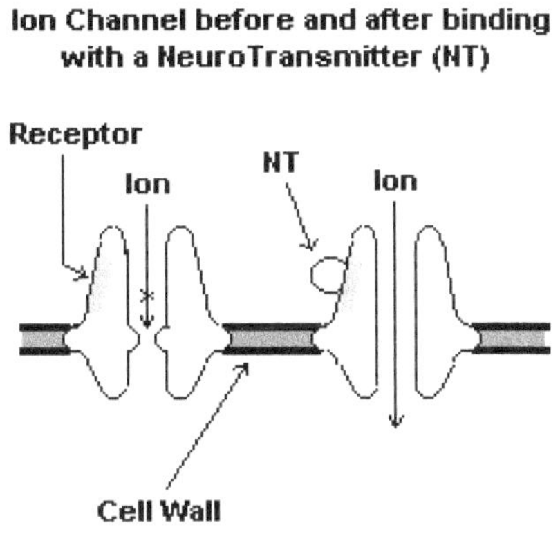

Fig 1.3.k Neurotransmitter e.g. – acetylcholine

1.3.11- Alkyl and Aryl Halides

Chlorine, iodine or bromine involved in alkyl halides tend to posses chemical reactivity as the halide ion are good leaving group. Due to this the drug possessing alkyl halide is easily capable of reacting with any of the nucleophilic group; targeting and making it covalently/permanently bonded i.e. an alkylation reaction (e.g. alkylation of enolates Fig 1.3.l) takes place. This reactivity is slightly problematic as the drugs are capable for alkylating wide range of macromolecules possessing nucleophillic group in it and also for amino group in nucleic acids and proteins. The problem in the reactivity can be moderated to a certain extent leading to severe side effects as selectivity is still a major problem. Therefore these drugs are not used in treatment of common diseases and are preserved for usage in life threatening diseases e.g. cancer. Alkyl group containing fluorides i.e. alkyl fluorides does not act as alkylating agents due to the presence of stronger C-F bond which cannot be easily broken. Fluorine due to its same size to that of proton is used to replace it but posses' different electronic properties. It has the ability to protect the molecules from undergoing metabolism.

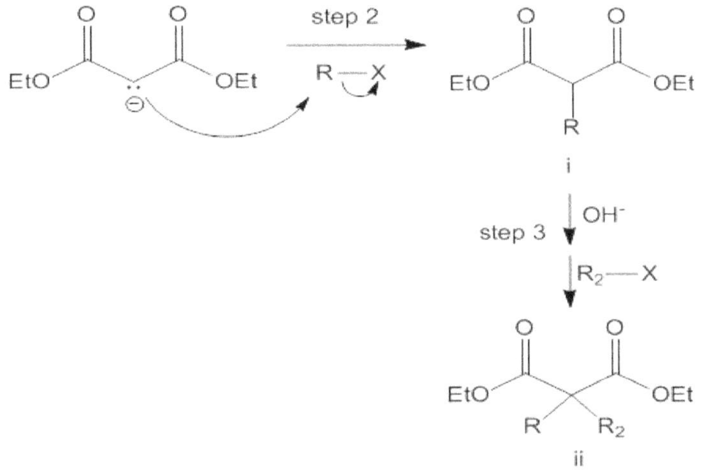

Fig 1.3.l alkylation of enolates

Aryl halides are not able to act as alkylating agents as the halogen substituents present in it are electron withdrawing groups affecting electron density, influencing binding nature of aromatic ring. Due to hydrophobic nature chlorine and bromine are favorable for interaction at binding site through hydrophobic pockets. Hence hydrogen bonding is not essential. Halogen substituents, halide ions are poor, strong hydrogen bond acceptors respectively.

1.3.12- Esters

An ester functional group is able to bind at the binding site only as a hydrogen bond acceptor. The carbonyl oxygen present in the functional group is more capable than alkoxy oxygen for acting as a hydrogen bond acceptor due to its less hindrance sterically and greater electron density. Fully synthesized equivalent ether can play an important role in testing carbonyl group. Esterases are the esters which can hydrolyze by metabolic enzymes in vivo. Due to this nature, the lead compounds containing esters (important for binding) may susceptible to problems decreasing the drug life-time in vivo. Ester groups are present in several drugs stabilizing itself towards metabolism mainly due to electronic or steric factors protecting esters. The hydrolysis of esters in the blood releasing the active drug is referred to as prodrug strategy. Aspirin exhibits an anti inflammatory action by inhibiting the cyclooxygenase enzyme (essential for the synthesis of prostaglandin). It also acts as acylating agent by covalently attaching to serine residue at COX active site (Fig 1.3.m). Aspirin is considered as a prodrug generating salicylic acid inhibiting enzyme by non covalent interactions.

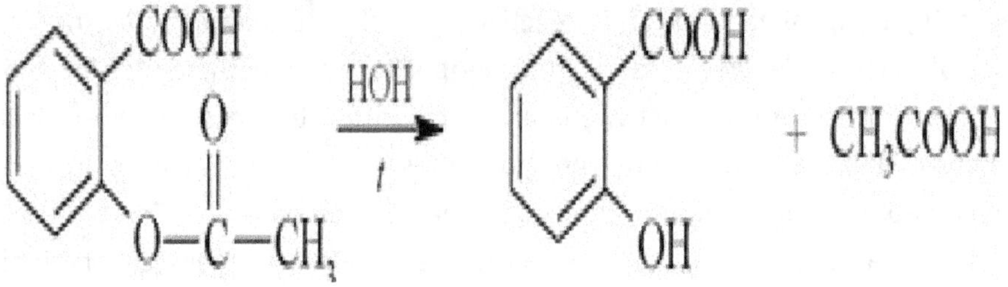

Fig 1.3.m aspirin- acylating agent

1.3.13- Carboxylic Acids

Carboxylic acid group is commonly present in many drugs it acts as both hydrogen bond acceptor and donor in various ways. It can also exist as carboxylate ion allowing the possibility of acting as hydrogen bond acceptor. Carboxylate ion for zinc ions acts as a good ligand, present in zinc metalloproteinases enzymes as a cofactor. Primary amides, primary alcohols, esters and ketones are the basic analogues synthesized and used for testing the carboxylic acid interactions (Fig 1.3.n). The above analogues are incapable to get ionized, indicating the importance of ionic bond at the time of loss of activity. Primary alcohol indicates that carbonyl oxygen participates in hydrogen bonding. In ester and ketone a hydroxyl group present in the carboxylic acid participates in hydrogen bonding. From lead compound ester and amide analogues can be synthesized directly but harsher conditions are required for reducing carboxylic acid to primary alcohol, therefore this analogue must be prepared through full synthesis. Ketone can also be prepared by full synthesis.

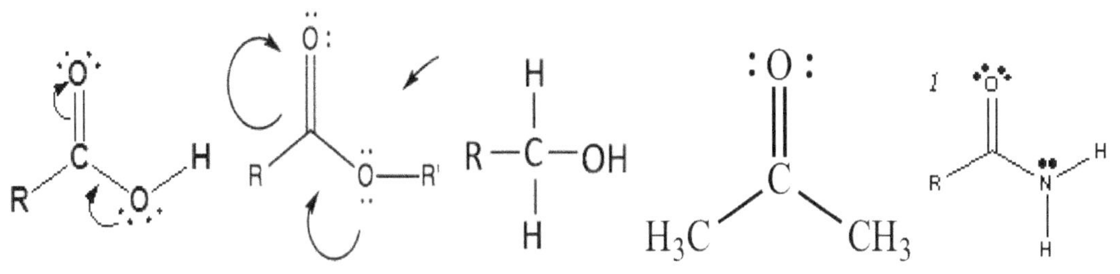

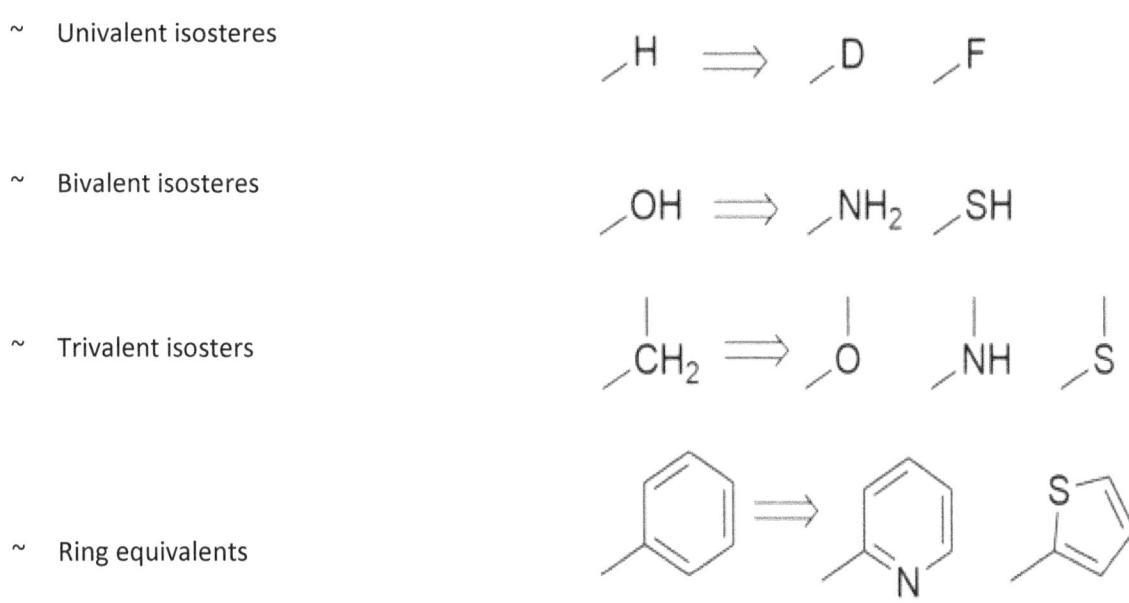

Carboxylic acid Ester primary alcohol ketone Primary amide

1.3.n Carboxylic acid- Analogues used for testing binding interactions.

1.3.14- Isosteres

Atoms or group of atoms possessing same valency in outer shell configuration with similar chemical and physical characteristics are referred to as isosteres (Fig 1.3.o).

- Univalent isosteres

- Bivalent isosteres

- Trivalent isosters

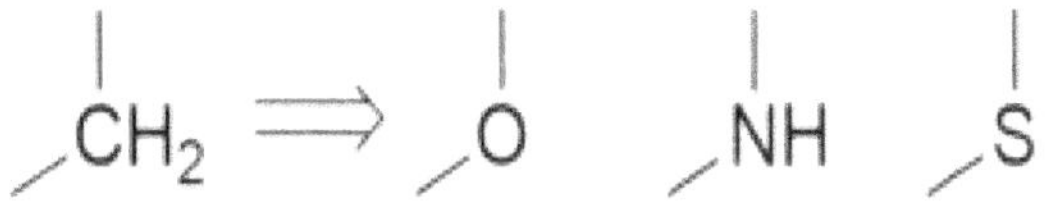

- Ring equivalents

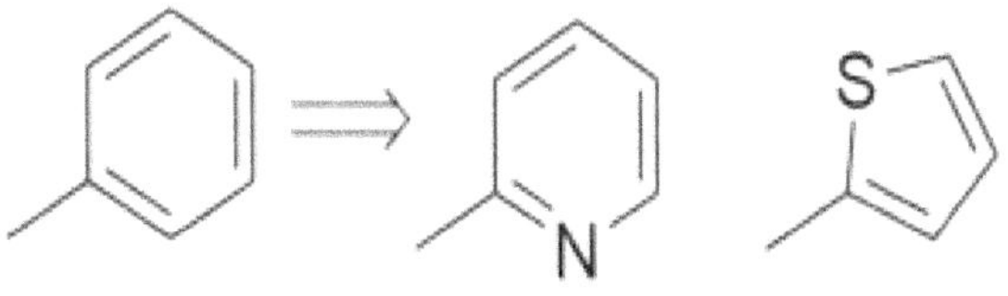

Fig 1.3.o classic isosteres

For hydroxyl group OH isosteres are CH3, NH2 and SH. For oxygen O isosteres are CH2 (dimethoxy isosteres (Fig 1.3.p), NH and S. isosteres function mainly in determination of the importance of a particular group in binding. By altering the groups the character can be effectively controlled. Replacement of CH2 by O makes a little difference in analogue size. Replacement shows a marked change in bonding, electronic distribution and polarity. Replacement of OH by larger SH influences steric factors and not the electronic character. In hydrogen bonding a particular group involved can be determined by the isosteric groups. For example consider OH replaced by CH3 eliminates the hydrogen bonding, whereas the replacement of OH by NH2 does not eliminate it.

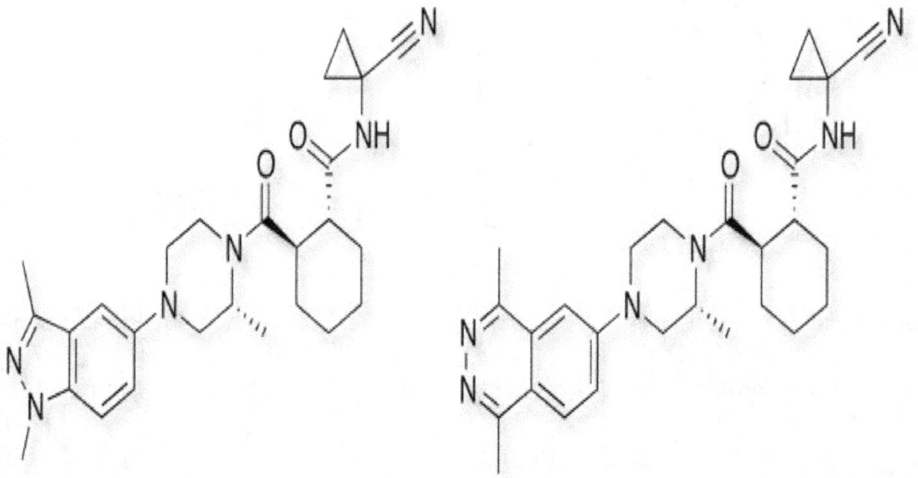

Fig 1.3.p Dimethoxy isosteres

An ether linkage is present in β blocker propranolol (Fig 1.3.q). OCH2 segment is replaced with CH=CH/CH2 CH2/SCH2 isosteres demolishes its activity completely. Whereas NHCH2 when replaced reduces yet retains its activity. These are indicative that ether oxygen is essential and is involved in hydrogen bonding of drug with the receptor.

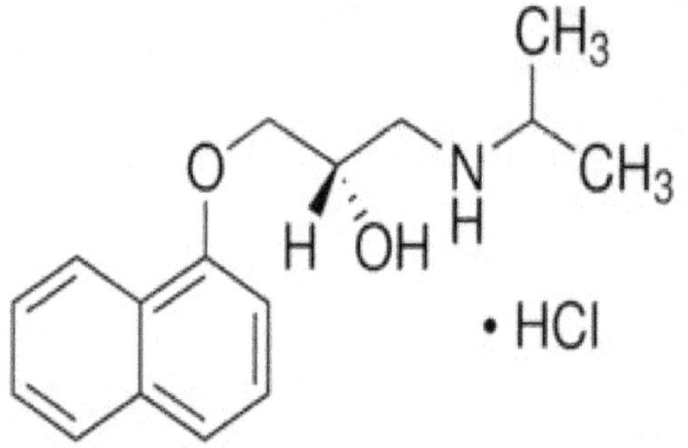

Fig 1.3.q propranolol

1.3.15- Heterocycles

In lead compounds large varieties of heterocyclic groups are present. These are the structures which contain hetero atoms (nitrogen, sulfur and oxygen) in their cyclic ring. Nitrogen containing heterocyclic compounds is common in nature. Heterocyclic compounds may either aromatic or aliphatic and are capable to bind and interact with variety of binding forces at the binding sites. When taken individually, the heteroatoms like sulfur, nitrogen and oxygen are capable to interact by hydrogen bonding at the binding site. Whereas overall compound can bind and interact through hydrophobic and van der waals forces.

In hydrogen bonding, aspects such as the orientation of ring and position of heteroatom are essential in determining the interaction stability (good or weak). Consider purine structure, it possesses 3 hydrogen bond acceptors and donors permitting 6 hydrogen bond interactions but in an ideal direction. In the purine ring vander waal interactions are possible above and below binding regions of ring system. Some heterocycles involves hydrogen binding intricate networks within binding site. Methotrexate, an anticancer drug can be considered as an example containing pteridine ring system (Fig 1.3.r) which basically interacts with binding site.

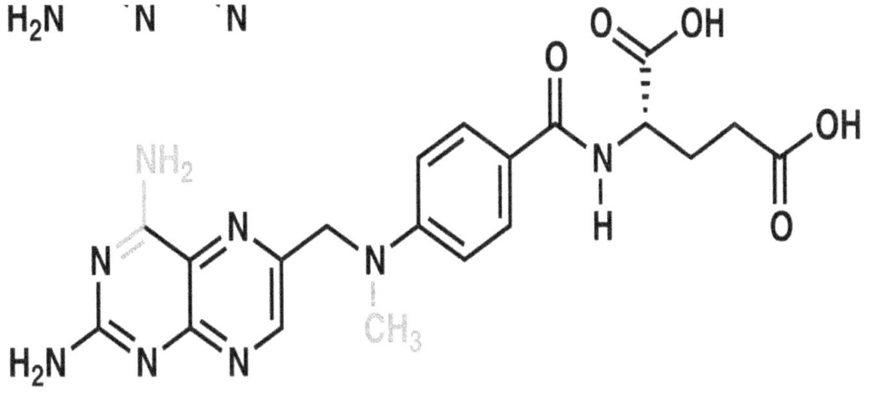

Fig 1.3.r methotrexate with pteridine ring system

If the heterocyclic ring is present in lead compound, analogues are to be synthesized exploring the necessity of these heteroatoms. Tautomers formed due to complication of heterocycles plays essential a role in determining DNA structure. Nucleic acid bases which are heterocyclic in nature are paired with double stranded helix constituting DNA structure. Guanine and cytosine are paired with three hydrogen bonds, and adenine and thymine are paired with two hydrogen bonds. Coplanar rings are involved in base pairing allowing ideal orientation for hydrogen bond acceptors and donors. The above arrangement leads to stacking of base pairs one above another, allowing the faces of base pairs for van der waal interactions. It is essential to determine the tautomers preferred by the heterocycles to ease the understanding of drugs interacting at the binding sites. A conjugated system is formed by hydrogen bond acceptors and donors of heterocyclic compounds. Enhancement of the hydrogen bond can be facilitated by bond cooperativity in conjugated system caused by polarization of electrons; this phenomenon is referred to as resonance-assisted hydrogen bonding possible for nucleic acid base pairs hydrogen bond acceptors and donors.

1.4 Drug Target Interaction- Testing Approach

After the investigation and studying of structure- activity relationships of compounds for their target binding interactions, biological testing is done which involves in vitro tests. In vitro tests such as isolated enzymes must be tested for inhibition studies, membrane bound receptors must be tested for binding studies in whole cells. These in vitro results are evaluated to know the importance of individual binding groups in drug target interactions. The in vivo tests can also be carried out but the results obtained are unclear and inapproximate as the activity of the drug is lost due to incapability to reach target site. in vivo tests are important in revealing functional groups essential for the drug to assist in flow in the body. These functional groups cannot be revealed through in vitro tests. in vitro tests were performed on natural benzophenones and their Structural diversity and bioactivities were studied (Fig 1.4). NMR spectroscopy is also an effective way to test the structure activity relationships of compounds.

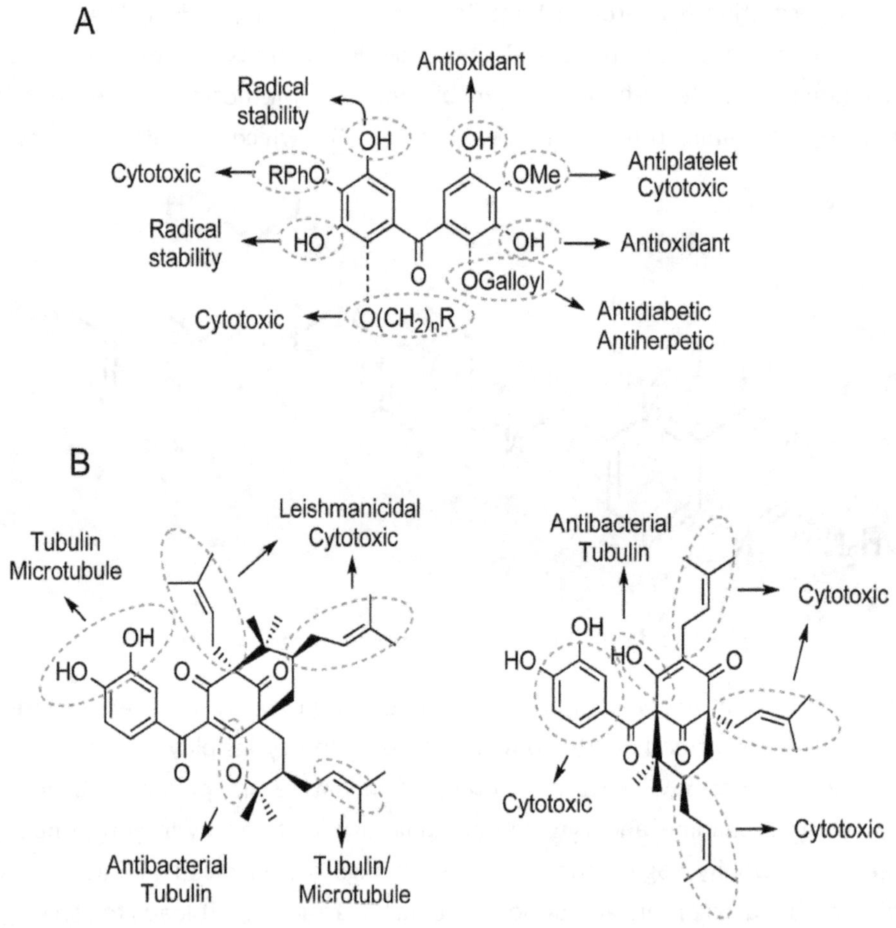

Fig 1.4 in vitro tests- Structural diversity and bioactivities of benzophenone

1.5 Pharmacophore Identification

After the establishment of groups which are responsible for drugs activity, next stage i.e. pharmacophore identification can be carried out. Pharmacophore is the specific part of a molecule responsible for biological/ pharmacological interaction of that molecule. Pharmacophores can also be defined as 'dummy bonds' using molecular modeling showing the bonds between nitrogen atom and centre of aromatic ring. Centroid is the dummy atom present at the centre of ring. Identification of the pharmacophore provides us with the binding groups which are important for activity, and also related to relative positions of molecules with respect to each other. Hypothetical drug glipine possess important binding groups like nitrogen atom, aromatic ring and two phenol groups. The pharmacophore structure can be given by structure I (2D- two dimensional), structure II (3 D- three dimensional) and structure III (specifies relative position in space). The nitrogen atom present in glipine is 5.036 A0 from center of its phenolic ring, lying at angle of 180. Displaying of the important groups connected by specific skeleton is not necessary rather it could have benefits not displaying it, as comparison among various different structural classes by 3D pharmacophores is easier and can show which compounds share a common pharmacophore. Bonding type pharmacophore is the more general 3D pharmacophore shown as structure III. Each functional group bonding characteristics are defined rather the entire structural group. Pharmacophore identification defines the group as the points in space. The aromatic ring is defined as the central point in ring namely centroid. Positions can be defined by joining the pints forming a pharmacophore triangle (e.g. cocaine pharmacophore triangle can be observed Fig 1.5.a). By this, molecules with the same pharmacophore and their binding interactions can be identified.

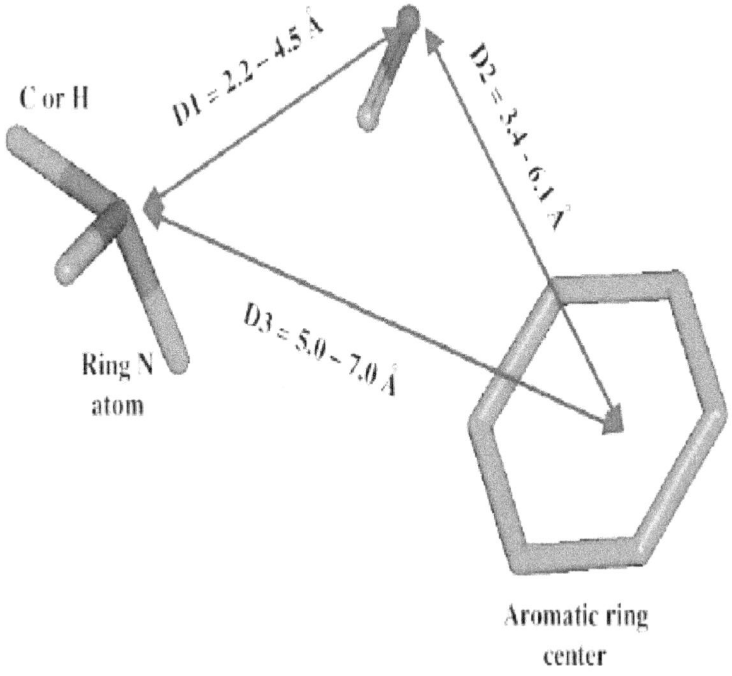

Fig 1.5.a e.g. Cocaine pharmacophore triangle

For differing functional groups phenol acting as hydrogen bond acceptor and donor can be used to achieve these interactions (e.g. two dissimilar molecules but have same pharmacophore model and are potent antimalarials Fig 1.5.b) with the aromatic ring of phenol participating in van der waals interactions, Amide if protonated can also act as ionic centre or hydrogen bond acceptor. 3D pharmacophores of rigid cyclic structures can easily be identified such as that of glipine. As the structure get more complex, possessing large no. of confirmations'/shapes with different binding groups at different positions. In these complex structures usually one conformation is at binding site is bounded and recognized, these conformations referred to as active conformations. Knowing the active conformations is essential for identifying the 3D pharmacophore. Various methods are there to achieve this. Various analogues of the compounds can be synthesized followed by their testing to study that whether their activity is retained or not. The target can be crystallized which is attached to the compound binding at the binding site. For determining the complex structure and its compound ligand-active conformation, x-ray crystallography can be used. For solving the active conformation of compounds which are isotopically labeled bounded to their active sites, progress is made in NMR spectroscopy.

Drawback- the pharmacophores are the interaction responsible part of molecule which can have unavoidable emphasis on their corresponding functional groups which are crucial for binding. This can be seen in some situations and not in some. Identifying the pharmacophore is common but rather shows effects on activity and exhibit poor binding. Through hydrophobic interactions and van der waal forces are involved in binding and interacting the overall skeleton to binding site. The effectiveness of the drugs can be determined based on the strength of interactions by means of 3D pharmacophore.

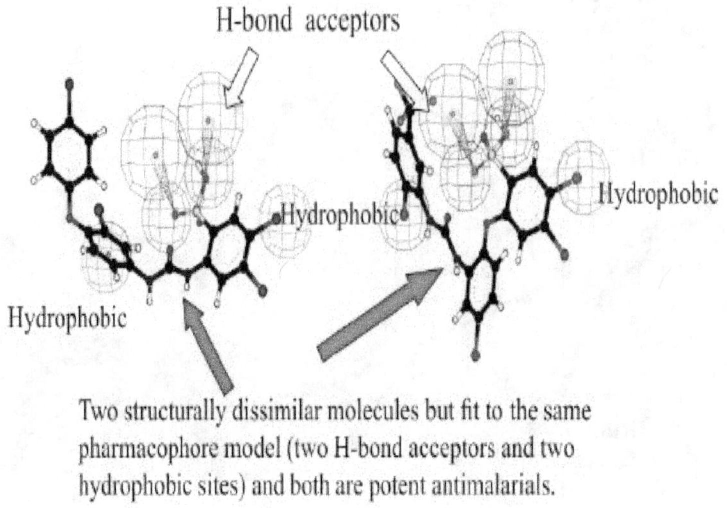

H-bond acceptors
Hydrophobic
Hydrophobic
Hydrophobic
Two structurally dissimilar molecules but fit to the same pharmacophore model (two H-bond acceptors and two hydrophobic sites) and both are potent antimalarials.

Fig 1.5.b different molecules having same pharmocophore showing similar antimalarial activity

1.6 Drug Optimization/Lead Identification and Drug Designing Strategies

After the identification of essential binding groups of lead compound and its pharmacophore, further analogues can be synthesized containing same pharmacophore. Lead compound has useful biological activity but very few of them are ideal, so it is required to synthesize analogues of that ideal lead compounds as most of them possess poor selectivity and are low active with many significant adverse effects. Synthesizing analogues of all lead compounds is difficult, rather than selecting the ideal ones with improved properties and synthesizing their analogues is an advantage. Strategies for optimizing drug-target interactions with higher activity and selectivity are considered.

1.6.1- Substituent Group: Variations

Easily accessible substituents are varied for tuning up the drug-target interactions.

Alkyl substituent's

In comparison with the other substituents, alkyl subsituents can more easily be varied. Consider compounds such as amides, amines, esters and ethers can easily be varied with alkyl substituents. The variation can be by means of removing the already present alkyl substituent and replacing it with the other. As a part of carbon skeleton the alkyl substituent cannot be removed in simple step but requires full synthesis to vary them. Alkyl substituents at binding site with hydrophobic pocket, depending on alkyl group length and bulk makes it t probe the pocket in terms of depth and width, t-butyl, isobutyl, isopropyl, butyl, propyl, ethyl and methyl are few of the examples for it (Fig 1.6.a).

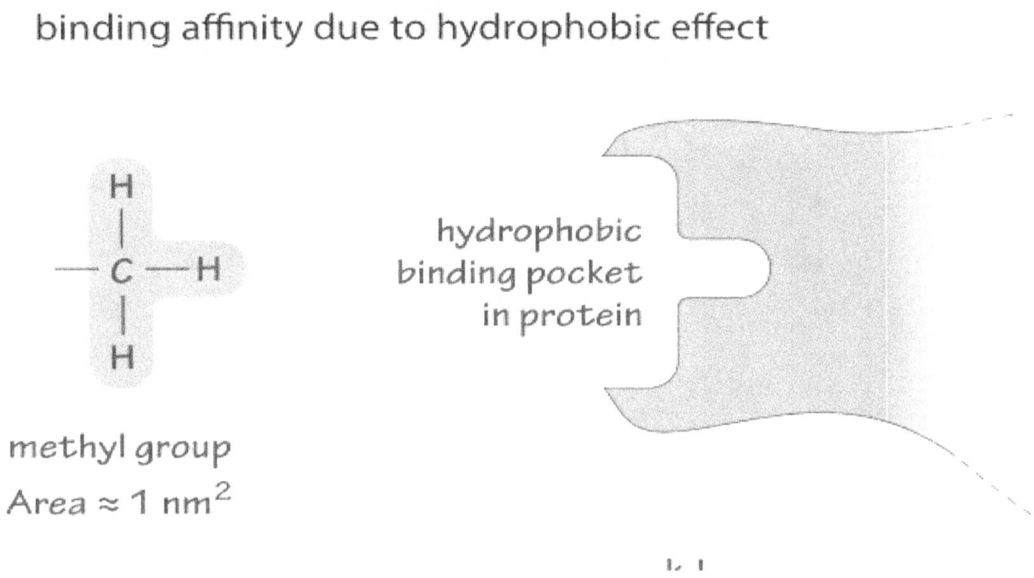

Fig 1.6.a binding of methyl group with hydrophobic pocket

Selectivity of the drug may also depend on the size of alkyl groups. Consider a drug interacting with different receptors; drug is prevented from binding by selective inhibition of targeted function, cutting down the adverse effects (Fig 1.6.b).

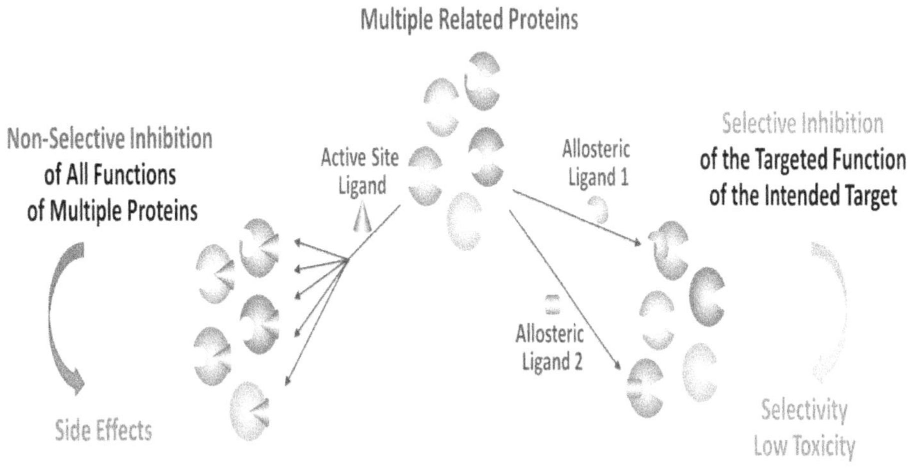

Fig 1.6.b Selective inhibition

For drug interacting with two receptors, prevention of attachment of drug to one of the receptor is done by the bulkier alkyl substituents reducing adverse effects (Fig 1.6.c).

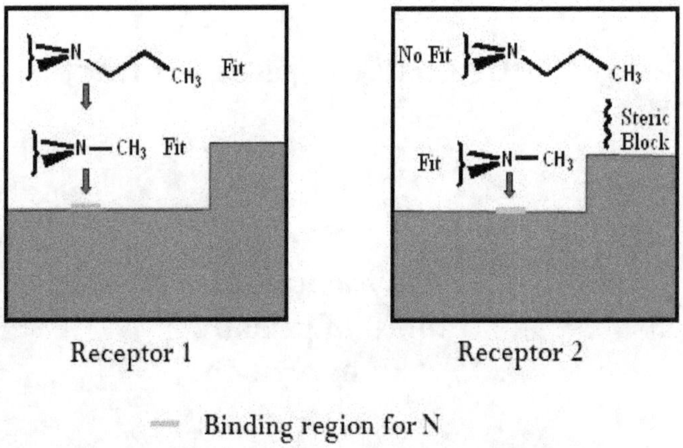

Fig 1.6.c usage of larger alkyl group to bring selectivity

For a compound adrenaline, an analogue isoprenaline is synthesized in which isopropyl group replaces methyl group. It results in selectivity of β-adrenergic receptors over α-receptors (Fig 1.6.d).

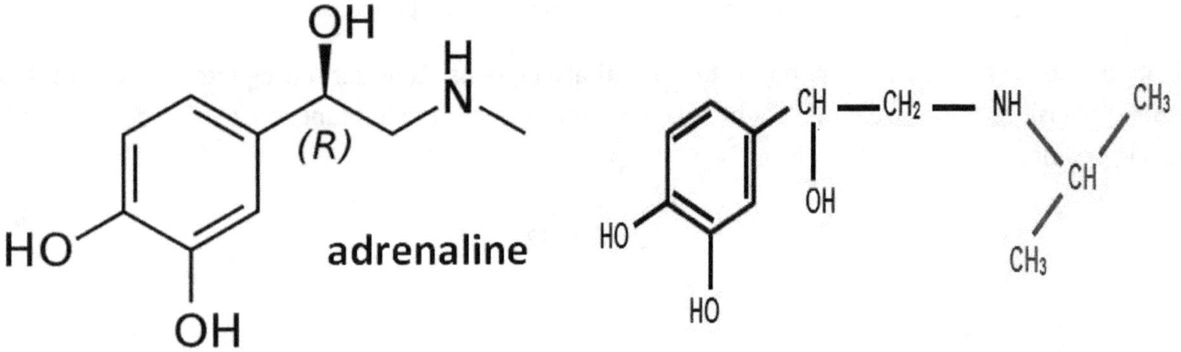

Adrenaline Isoprenaline

Fig 1.6.d Adrenaline and its analogue Isoprenaline

Aromatic substituent's

Drug containing aromatic ring provides with the benefit of varying substituents at any position finding better binding interactions with increased activity (Fig 1.6.e). From a series of benzopyrans, the one with best anti arrhythmic activity was found with sulfonamide substituent positioned at the 7 position of aromatic ring e.g. 4-Oxospiro[benzopyran-2,4'-piperidines] (Fig 1.6.f). Substituent variation at different positions may affect the substituent at another position. For example nitro group which is electron withdrawing when placed at para position inspite of meta position effects the basicity more significantly of an aromatic amine (Fig 1.6.g). The amine will become a weaker base when nitro group is placed at para position and makes it less liable to protonate decreasing its ability to undergo ionic bonding with ionic binding groups decreasing activity at binding site.

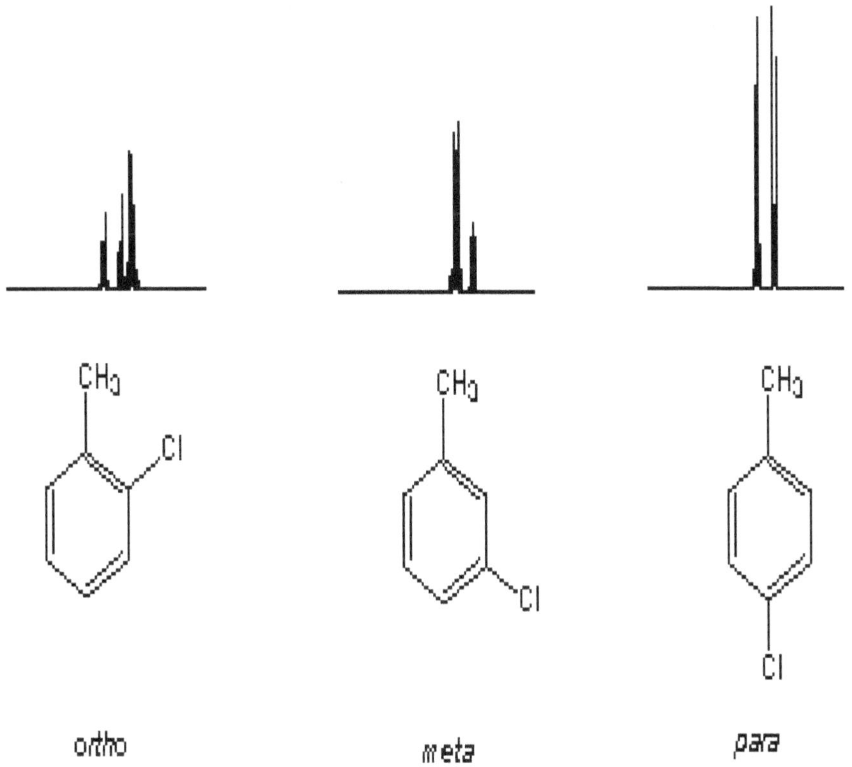

Fig 1.6.e Varying substituents at aromatic ring

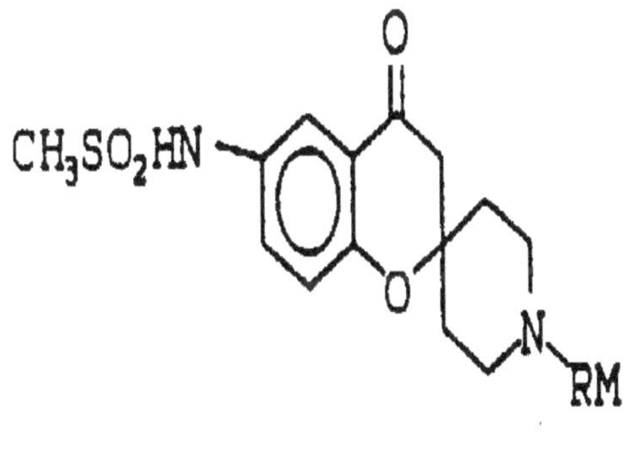

Fig 1.6.f benzopyrans (4-Oxospiro[benzopyran-2,4'-piperidines])

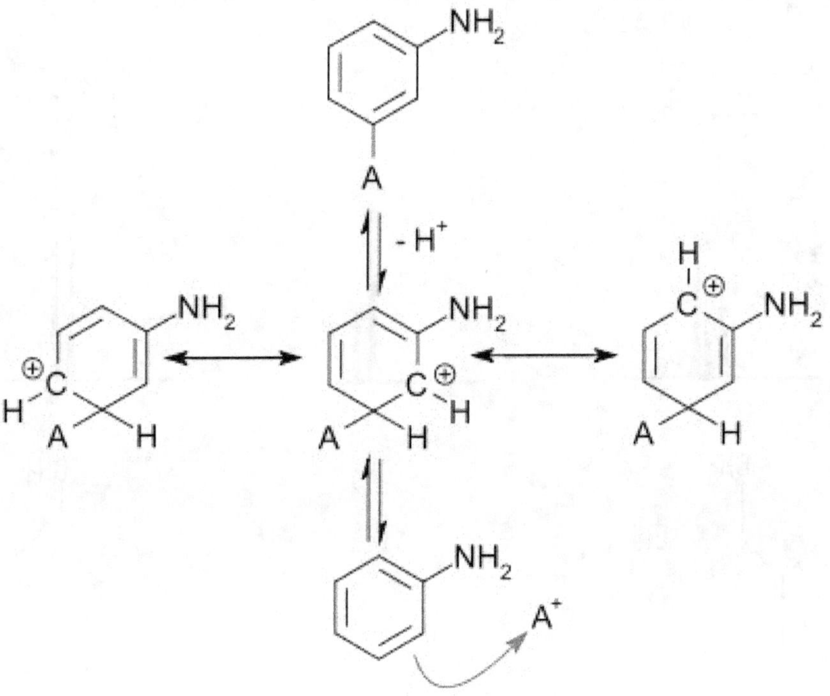

Meta directing reaction (inductive electron withdrawing)

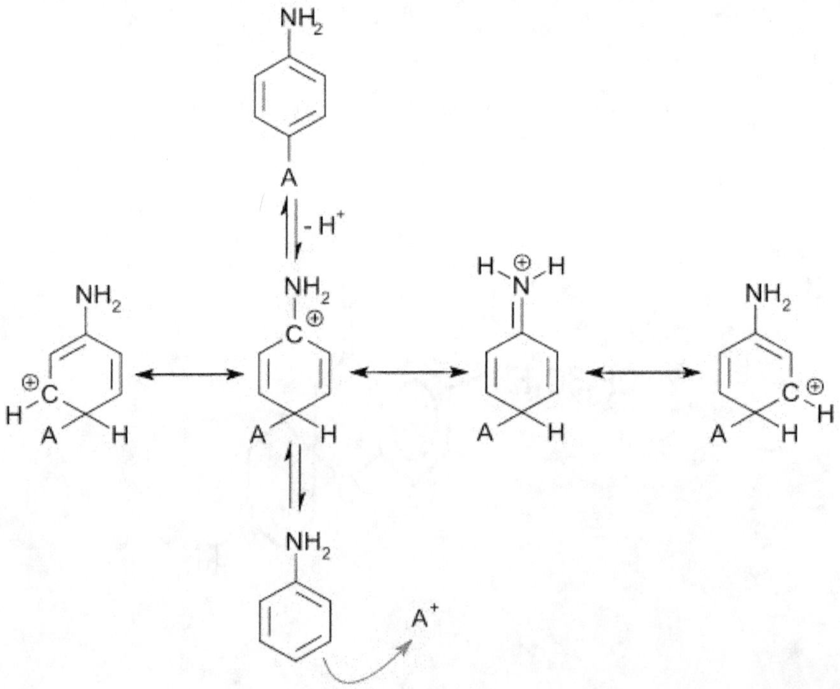

Para directing reaction (resonance and inductive effect contributes for electron withdrawing effect)

Fig 1.6.g Electronic effects produced due to different substitution patterns

If the structures possess an ideal substitution pattern, then only the substituents attaching to it are varied. Steric, electronic and hydrophobic characteristics differ with each substituent, varying the effect at binding sites and their activities. For example when cholro substituent i.e. an electron withdrawing substituent replaces a methyl substituent, then the activity may be improved (Fig 1.6.h).

$$\underset{\textbf{Methane}}{CH_4} + Cl_2 \xrightarrow[-HCl]{\text{Diffused Sunlight}} \underset{\textbf{Chloromethane}}{CH_3Cl}$$

$$CH_3Cl + Cl_2 \xrightarrow[-HCl]{} \underset{\textbf{Dichloromethane}}{CH_2Cl_2}$$

$$CH_2Cl_2 + Cl_2 \xrightarrow[-HCl]{} \underset{\textbf{Trichloromethane}}{CHCl_3}$$

$$CHCl_3 + Cl_2 \xrightarrow[-HCl]{} \underset{\textbf{Tetrachloromethane}}{CCl_4}$$

Fig 1.6.h chloro substituent replacing methyl substituent

Straight forward chemistry is involved in these substituents variation procedures. So analogues are synthesized for development of a novel drug. The alkyl and aromatic substituents variations are then open up for quantitative structure activity relationship studies.

1.6.2- Structure Extension

Another functional group addition to the lead compound is referred to as the strategy of extension. The extension is done to probe the extra binding interactions of the drug with its target. Lead compounds possess essential functional groups for interacting with binding regions and are capable of fitting. For lead compounds, it is not possible to interact with every binding region available to the compound. For example consider there are four binding regions available for the interaction, but lead compound is capable to interact with three binding regions only and the fourth one is left. To compensate the fourth one with binding interactions and to increase its activity additional functional groups are added (Fig 1.6.i). Finding of the additional hydrophobic regions by adding alkyl/aryl alkyl groups at the binding site is referred to as Extension tactics. These groups can be added in the form of phenols, alcohols, carboxylic acid and amines to the functional groups present in the drug. To increase additional hydrogen bonding/ ionic interactions, other functional groups can also be added.

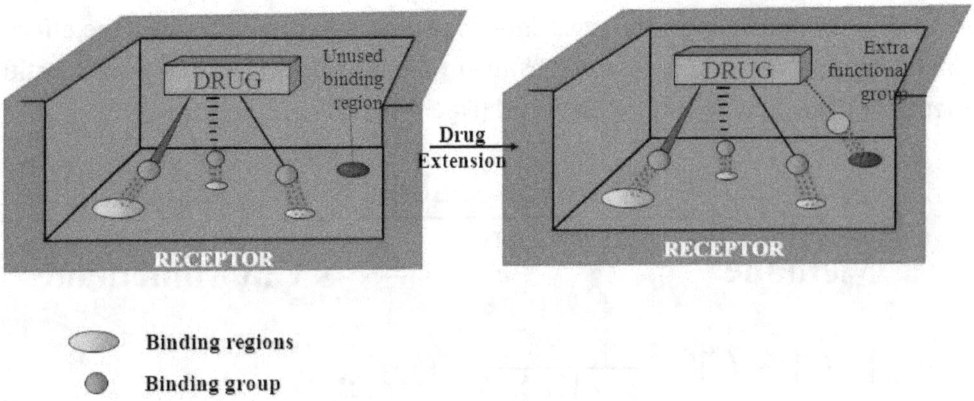

Fig 1.6.i Drug is extended to compensate the fourth binding group

An agonist can be converted into antagonist with the help of extension strategies. This can usually happen when a binding interaction is not used by natural substrate/agonist. A different overall binding interaction is resulted leading to production of antagonist activity over the agonist. Many active adrenergic agents and analogues of morphine are produced successfully with the help of extension tactics. The activity and selectivity can also be improved with the help of extension tactics, like that of protein kinase inhibitor and imatinib.

1.6.3- Extension or Contraction of Chain

In some cases the drug consists of chain linked together with two binding groups, in which there is no ideal chain structure for interaction with binding site. Therefore, in such cases the tactics used for chain length to shortened or lengthened can be tried to improve the interaction far possible (Fig1.6.j).

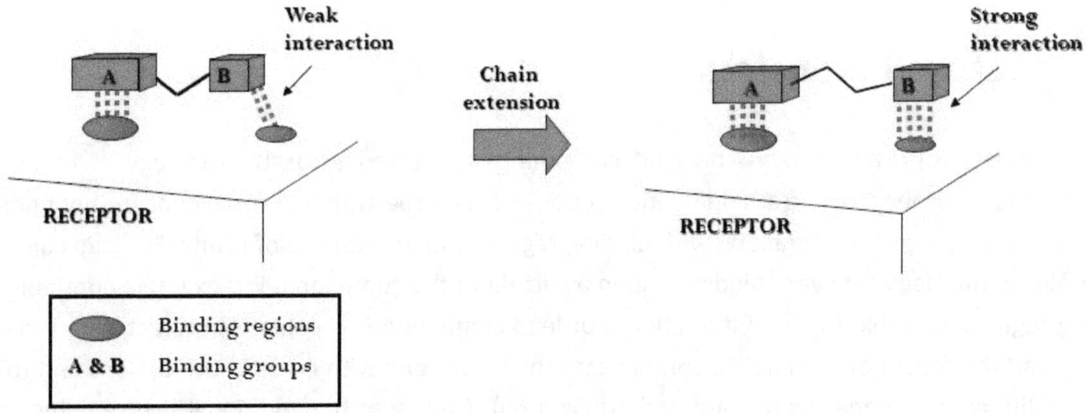

Fig 1.6.j chain contraction and extension

1.6.4- Extension or Contraction of Ring

For drugs containing more than one ring essential for its binding, it is worthy to synthesize the drug analogues in which the expansion or contraction of these rings takes place. The principle of expansion or contraction of the rings is same pattern that of involved in substituent variations of an aromatic ring. The expansion or contraction of the rings present more than one in a drug can bring them into newer and better positions in relation to one another and mat enhance the interaction rate with the particular essential regions/rings at their binding sites (Fig 1.6.k).

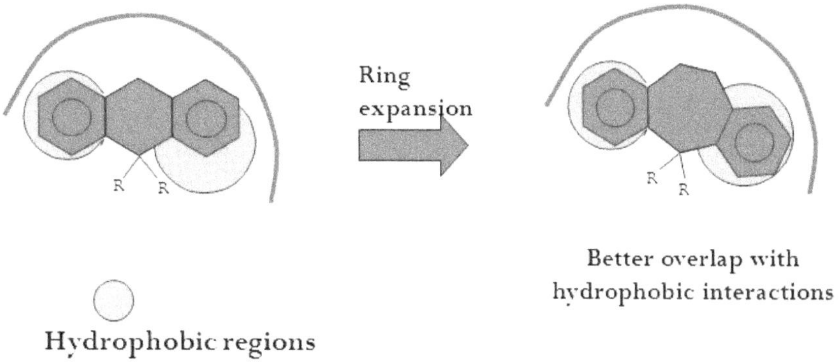

Fig 1.6.k Ring expansion aiding better hydrophobic interactions

Variations in the ring size aid the substituents with better positions for binding to occur. For example consider cilazaprilat, an anti-hypertensive drug and ACE inhibitor exhibit bicyclic structure I with promising activity (Fig 1.6.l). In this one amide and two carboxylate groups were the essential binding groups. By performing expansion and contraction of the ring, clizaprilat was found to exhibit the best interaction at binding site.

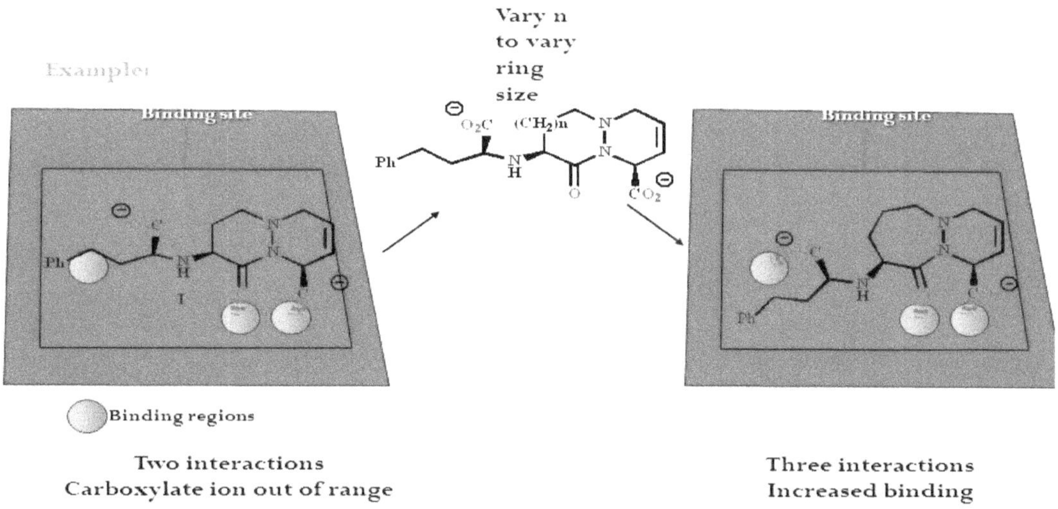

Fig 1.6.l Clizaprilat developed by ring expansion

1.6.5- Variations in the Ring

The replacement of the original aromatic or the heterocyclic ring with different sizes of heteroatomic ring and differently positioned heteroatoms is the widely used strategy bringing variations in the ring. Several NSAIDs- non steroidal anti-inflammatory agents with central 1,2-biaryl substituted ring are reported. In various pharmaceutical companies ring variation strategy is used for the production of wide range of active compounds (Fig 1.6.m).

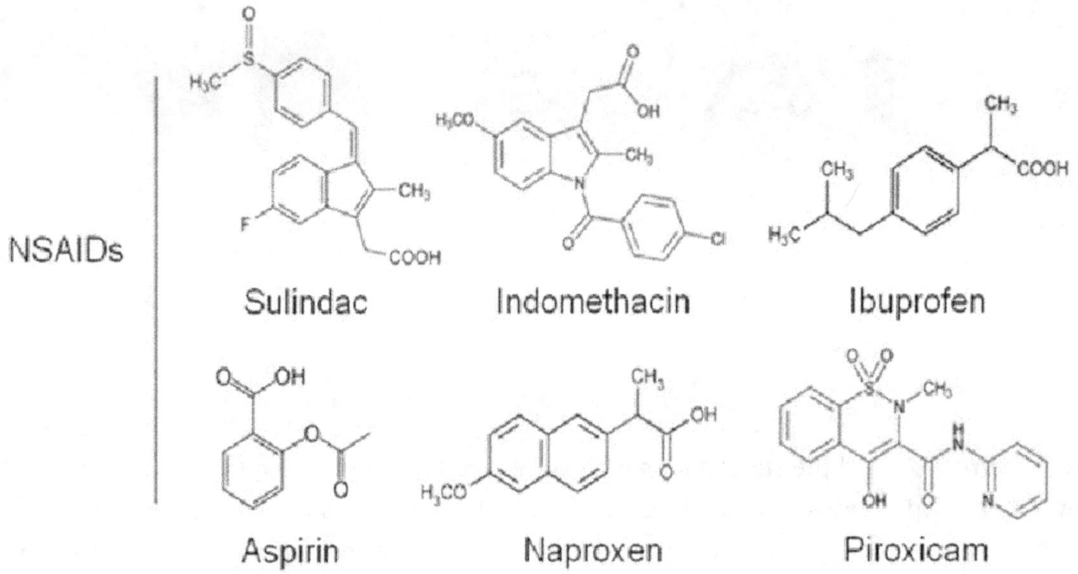

Fig 1.6.m Non-steroidal anti-inflammatory drugs

The strategy used is avoiding the patent restrictions making the similar changes with other one. But various activity, selectivity improvements are noticed with reduced adverse effects. Consider an antifungal agent I found in both fungal cells and humans acting against enzymes present in them. In this antifungal agent the 1,2,4-triazole ring replacing the imidazole ring giving UK 46245 showed enhanced selectivity against fungal enzyme (Fig 1.6.n).

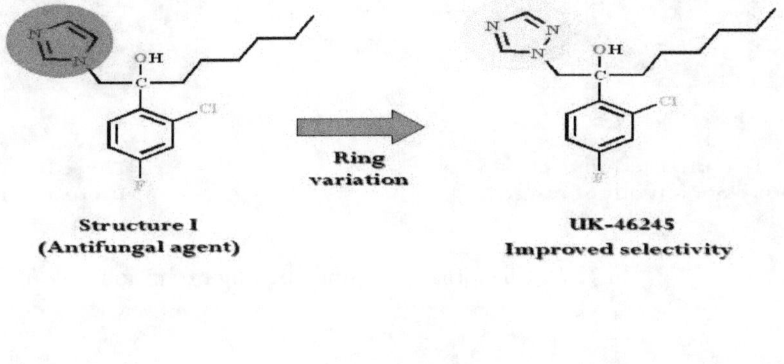

Fig 1.6.n Variations in ring for development of UK 46245

The advantage of this strategy is the upcoming of ability to undergo hydrogen bonding interactions with available binding sites. For example consider the pyridine ring replacing the aromatic ring in lead compound led to the production of Nevirapine drug with potent antiviral properties (Fig 1.6.o).

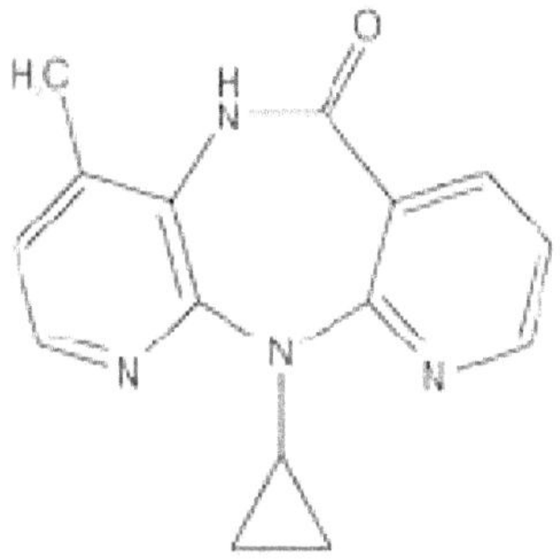

NEVIRAPINE

Fig 1.6.o Nevirapine

1.6.6- Extension of Ring by Ring Fusion

Interaction with the binding site and selectivity of the drug can be increased by ring fusion i.e. extension of ring. In developing β blockers, one of the major advances is the aromatic ring replacement with pronethaol (naphthalene ring) in adrenaline resulting in production of compound which was able to easily distinguish α,β-adrenaline similar receptors (Fig 1.6.p).

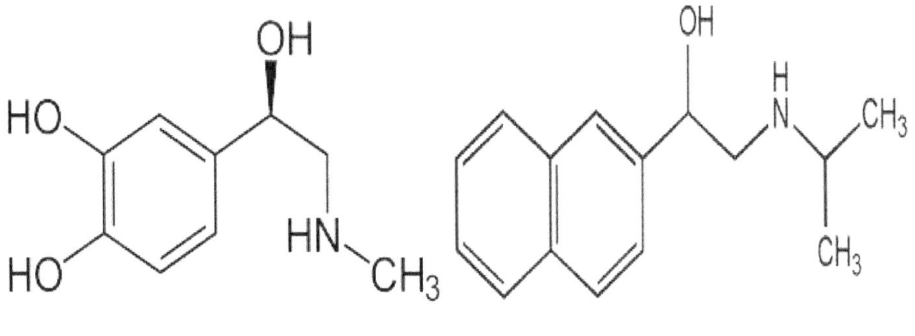

Adrenaline pronethalol

Fig 1.6.p structures of adrenaline and pronethalol

α-receptor has smaller vander waal binding area when compared to that of β-receptor which has the ability to strongly interact with pronethalol than adrenaline. It can also be because of the naphthalene ring which is perfect for β-receptor and is big sterically for α-receptor.

1.6.7- Isosteres and Bioisosteres

In the drug design isosteres are used for varying the molecule character in rational way in relation with characteristics such as the size, electronic distribution, polarity and its bonding. The essentiality of the size in interaction can be determined by the isosteres and the electronic factors can be determined by others. As hydrogen and fluorine are of same size, the isosteres for hydrogen is considered as fluorine. As fluorine is highly electronegative, it varies electronic properties of the compound without a slight change in steric nature. The enzymatic reaction can be disrupted by replacing enzymatically liable hydrogen with the help of fluorine. In this case the breakage of C-F bonds gets difficult. 5-fluorouracil an antitumor drug has capability to interact with target enzyme of normal substrate uracil due to slight change from it. In this during the enzyme mechanism the hydrogen is completely lost and enzyme catalyzed reaction is entirely disrupted. For replacing functional groups in drug design various non- classic isosteres can be used. Non-classic isosteres are the one which are opposite to classic isosteres having same physical and chemical characteristics but doesn't obey their steric and electronic properties.

Classic and non-classic isosteres in drug design are together referred to as bioisostere. These are the groups which are capable to retain the desired biological activity despite of replacing another group in it. They usually replace the functional groups essential for binding but led to problems. Consider thiourea group in early histamine group acts as an essential group but leads to severe toxic effects. Bioisosteres replaces and retains the histamine antagonism allowing essential binding interactions avoiding toxicity. Every bioisostere is specific for certain compounds and their binding sites. Replacing bioisostere in place of functional group doesn't guarantee retaining the drug activity. The use of bioisostere increases the binding interactions and its selectivity replacing the problematic group hence retaining the actual activity of the drug. For amide the bioisostere used is pyrrole ring. Replacement of problematic group in sulpiride; dopamine antagonist showed increased activity and selectivity of D3-receptor (dopamine) over D2-receptor (Fig 1.6.q). These agents exhibited anti-psychotic property lacking adverse effects.

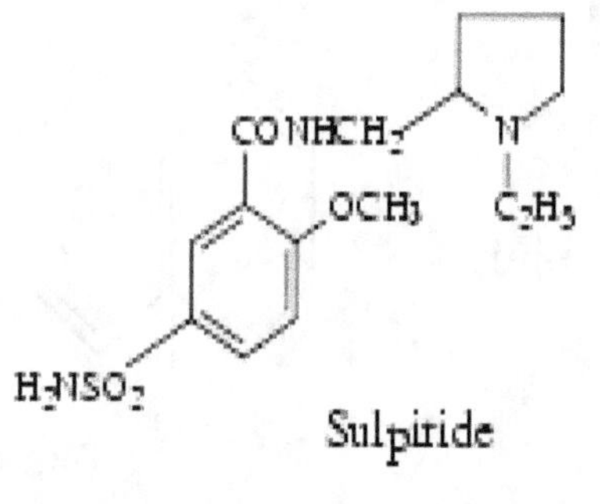

Fig 1.6.q Structure of dopamine antagonist

The replacement of problematic group with that of bioisostere often enhances and aids in extra binding interactions of the drug with its binding site. for example increased activity was observed when carboxylic acid was synthesized using N-acylsulfonamide as an bioisostere inducing increased possibilities for hydrogen bonding/van der waal interactions too occur at the binding site.

For designing of the transition-state analogues in drug design, special type of isosteres such as transition-state isosteres are used. They usually inhibit the enzymes which causes the enzymatic reactions. In this reaction a substrate is required to pass through the transition state by getting activated before it forms a product. The design of the transition state is focused mainly for drug designing rather than the substrate/product structure. The stability of the transition state enables the transition state isosteres to mimic essential features of transition state. The unstable compounds can be rendered stable by the transition state isosteres.

1.6.8- Structure Simplification

The natural lead compounds which are complex in nature are usually simplified by the structure simplification strategy. After the identification of essential groups, non essential groups can be discarded easily without the loss of activity. The functional groups which are not essential and do not form a pharmacophore are removed. The carbon skeleton is simplified and asymmetric centers are removed. In Glipine, a hypothetical natural product the important groups are known and with this the simpler compounds are aimed to synthesize (Fig 1.6.r). The pharamcophore is retained in this process.

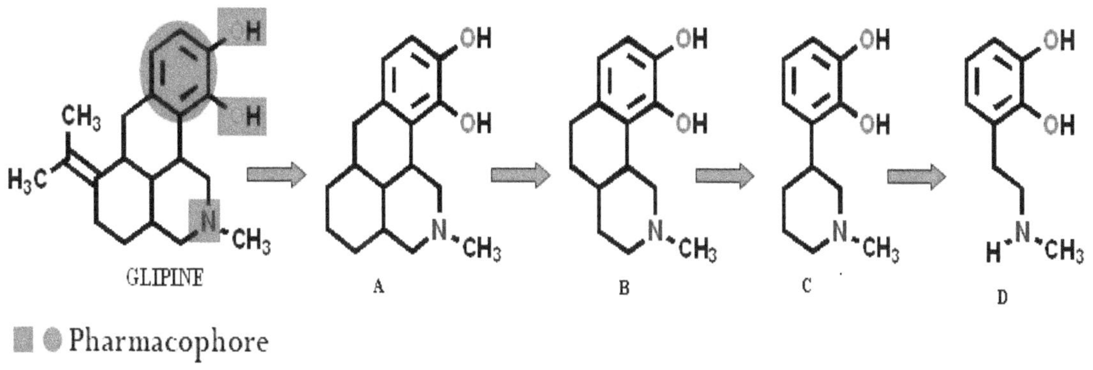

Fig 1.6.r Simplification of Glipine (analogues are synthesized)

Racemate making is the cheapest and easiest method to synthesize chiral drug. The activity and adverse effects of the obtained enantiomers are then tested as each of them possesses different characteristics. The pure enantiomer is preferred over the racemates which is usually extracted by enantiomers separating of the racemic mixture/asymmetric synthesis.

Asperlicin a microbial metabolite has been simplified retaining the indole and benzodiazepine skeleton, by simplification technique to devazepide (Fig 1.6.s).

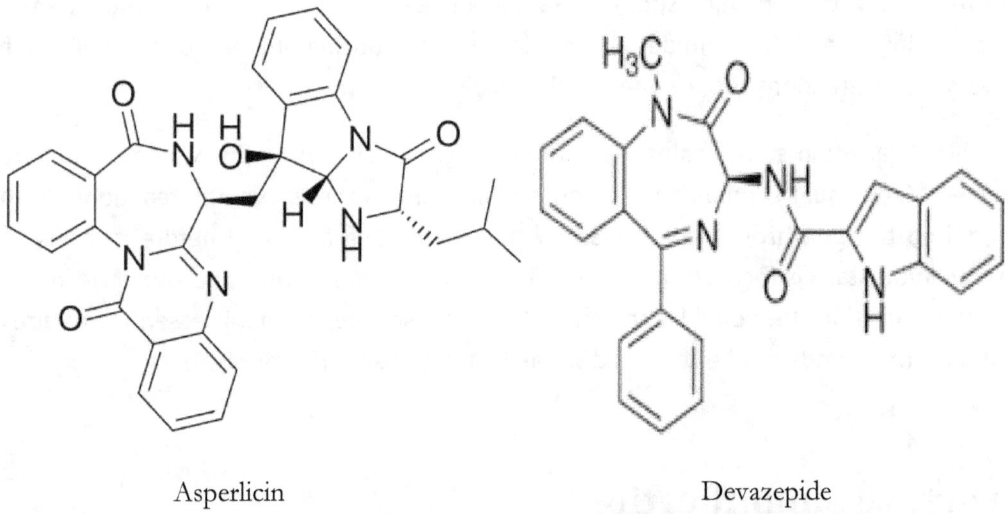

Fig 1.6.s Simplification of asperlicin to devazepide

The perfect simplification of the structure refers to the drug designed eliminating almost entire or some asymmetric centers from the compound making it advantageous in all aspects. For example consider mevinolin; cholesterol lowering agents possess eight asymmetric centers. Second generation cholesterol lowering agent is developed with enhanced activity having far fewer asymmetric centers.

Asymmetric carbon centers can be removed by various tactics such as nitrogen replacing carbon center is effective. Introduction of symmetry in the compound which has none is another tactic used. The simplified structures have the advantage of been synthesized in an easier, quicker and cheaper way in the pharmaceutical laboratories. The naturally occurring lead compounds are difficult to synthesize artificially. By eliminating functional groups various adverse effects are reduced. Oversimplification can also be disadvantageous as simpler molecules are capable to bind to their targets directly yielding different effects, reduced activity and selectivity with increased adverse effects. Simplification should be done in stages retaining desired activity at individual stages.

1.6.9- Structure Rigidification

Increasing the activity of the drug and reducing its adverse effects can be obtained effectively by the process of rigidification. Consider neurotransmitter as an example for understanding the achievement of rigidification. Neurotransmitter is a simple and a flexible molecule. Large no. of conformations/shapes can be obtained by bond rotation. The active confirmation is the first conformation in the structure i.e. conformation I recognized by the receptor. The inactive conformation i.e. conformation II is ionized having the ionic group far from center effecting the interaction, thus is inactive with model receptor binding site. A receptor capable of binding with inactive conformation II is possible to exist. In spite of been very flexible, the human body is incapable to release it near the binding target receptor site. They are also inactivated soon, preventing the neurotransmitter to bind with other receptors. The above case is not seen for drugs. The drugs have the ability to travel throughout the body and interact with any receptor able to accept it. If the drugs are highly flexible they go and interact with many receptors leading to severe adverse effects. Therefore excess flexible drugs are not suitable for oral medications/bioavailability (Fig 1.6.t).

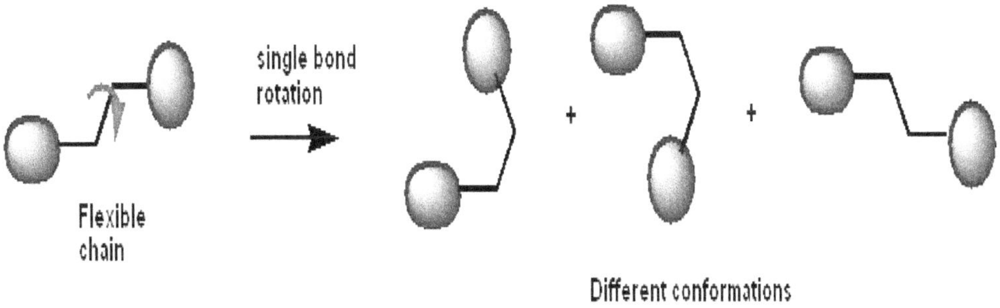

Fig 1.6.t Excess flexibility results in different conformations

To prevent the drug from attaining various shapes and conformations, the molecules are locked to form rigid structure/conformation usually referred to as rigidification. Acyclic pentapeptide is also rigidified using rigidification strategy. Strategy of rigidification is to prevent unrequired interactions of drugs with receptor and to prevent adverse effects. This strategy must also enhance the activity making the drug rigid for locking with target receptor and forming active conformation fitting the drug perfectly in its target. Incorporation of flexible skeleton in the drug is a common method to lock a conformation and the analogues synthesized for such drugs must be rigid (Fig 1.6.u).

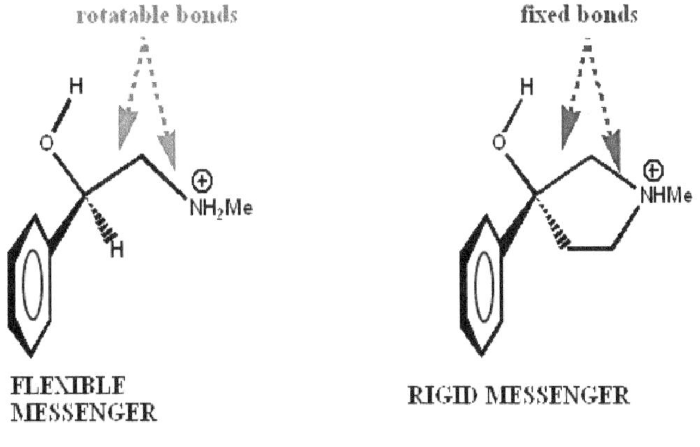

Fig 1.6.u Structure rigidification (locking of bonds)

For development of cilazapril; an anti-hypertensive agent from captopril rigidification tactics are involved. Rigidification simply doesn't mean the locking of rotatable bond in the structure ring, a side chain which is flexible should be rigidified partially with the incorporation of functional double bonds (=bond, aromatic ring, alkyne or amide). Apart from advantageous it also has few disadvantages like; its synthesis is more complicated.

No guarantee is given to retain the active conformation by rigidification. By rigidification it can also be possible to obtain a compound locked as inactive conformation. As the target sites are also prone to mutations, the changes occurring may lead to alteration in the shape of binding site making the drug incapable to bind.

1.6.10-Conformational Blockers

The strategy involved in rigidification tactics restricts the conformations possible for a compound. Conformational blockers is the another tactic having the effects of that of rigidification tactics. In certain cases there are compounds to which the addition of a single substituent hinders the free rotation of compounds. Consider dopamine (D3) antagonist I in which the addition of methyl substituent results in antagonist II with a dramatic reduction in its affinity. Bad steric clash occurs between the proton situated at ortho position at neighboring ring and methyl group preventing the rings to lie on the same plane. The rotation between the two neighboring rings at bond level is no further possible and attains a conformation at which both lie at an angle in the same plane with respect to each other. Structure I allows the free rotation of bonds between the rings attaining an active conformation in which the structures are coplanar. The role of the conformational blocker at this stage is to reject the active conformation. 4-methylhistamine, serotonin antagonist and imatinib (increased activity as well as selectivity between target sites) are the few examples used as conformational blockers (Fig 1.6.v). Rigidification is aided with intermolecular hydrogen bonding, stabilizing conformations e.g. kinase inhibitor SU 5416.

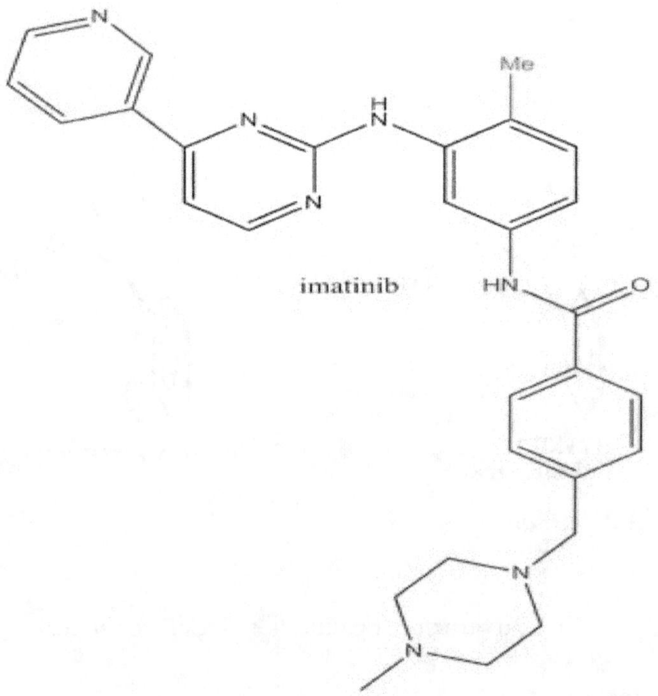

Fig 1.6.v Conformational blocker- Imatinib

1.6.11- Drug Designing and Molecular Modeling Based on Structure

The drug designing traditional strategies were discussed without the knowledge of target structure these strategies were carried out, resulting in the information essential for target binding site. An essential binding group present in a drug is an indicative of the presence of complementary binding region on the receptor/enzyme. X-ray crystallography plays an essential role in determining the structure if the macromolecular target is isolated and then crystallized, but x-ray crystallography is unable to detect the binding site present. So, it is beneficial to use an antagonist/inhibitor for crystallizing the protein, which is bounded at the binding site. Then it gets easier for x-ray crystallography for determining structure, which later can be downloaded using a computer. Then the ligand is identified using molecular modeling software and identifying the binding site. Essential binding interactions can be identified by measuring the distance between ligand (atoms of ligand) and binding site (atoms at binding site). After the above procedure, using a silico the ligand is removed from the binding site, followed by the insertion of novel lead compounds in silico to observe its fitness at the binding site. The binding site is observed and regions left vacant by the binding site are observed and are used by the medicinal chemist to undergo various modifications in the structure for designing a new drug. The newly synthesized drug is tested for its biological activity. If the drug synthesized is active then crystallization of the target protein is done, followed by the tests performed by x-ray crystallography and molecular modeling. The complex structure and its binding site are identified. The entire approach is referred to as structure based drug design. Based on the knowledge of binding site alone, the designing of the novel drug slightly related to structure based drug design is known as de novo drug design. Many novel lead compounds were designed using de novo/structure based drug design. If the target of the lead compound is left unidentified then the structure based drug design is of no use, if identified it's not necessary that it may get crystallize. It can be seen in membrane bound proteins. This can be overcome by finding out the protein similar to that of target protein followed by crystallization and is then studied using x-ray crystallography. The information obtained in terms of structural and mechanistic from protein analogues is used for the designing of the target proteins. The compounds differing in nature but are capable to interact with similar target can be studied using molecular modeling. Pharmacophores are used for comparison of these structures, making the novel design possessing similar pharmacophores. Novel lead compounds can be identified using the searched pharmacophores from compound databanks. Molecular modeling has various advantages in the medicinal chemistry but there are few drawbacks. Molecular modeling tackles only a part i.e. designing of an effective drug, of a huge problem. Chemist may design a product which perfect with terms of binding t target receptor and its activity but is unable to synthesize or reach target site in human body, it is of no use.

1.6.12- NMR Drug Designing

NMR spectroscopy is an effecting way of designing lead compounds, focusing mainly to design a potent lead compound. Drug design mainly focuses on optimizing the lead compound after its discovery. NMR spectroscopy firstly involves the epitopes optimization to maximize binding interactions. Secondly, these epitopes are linked t form a final product.

The non crystallizing target proteins are identified using the NMR spectroscopy and then the results are studied by X-ray crystallography. After the identification of the structure, molecular modeling techniques are carried out for designing of drugs.

1.6.13- Groping in Dark

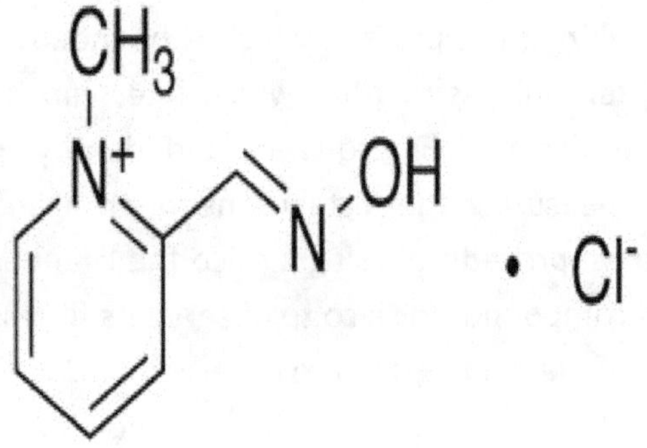

Pralidoxine

Now a day's rational drug designing is carried out for designing drugs but it doesn't mean that the role of hard working medicinal chemists is not eliminated. In the market most drugs present are developed from rational design mixture, trials and luck. ACE inhibitors, HIV protease inhibitors, thymidylate synthase inhibitors, neuraminidase inhibitors, cimetidine and pralidoxine are few of the drugs developed by rational drug design but are still minority (Fig 1.6.w).

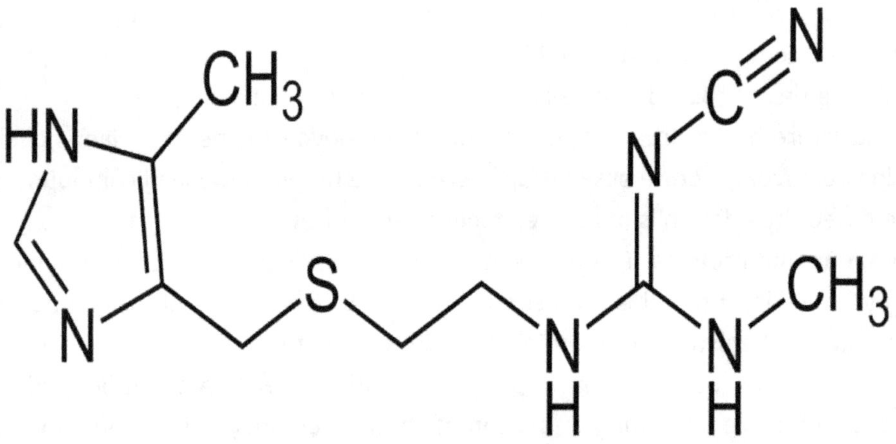

Cimetidine

Fig 1.6.w Structure of pralidoxine and cimetidine

Literature of the compounds is highly beneficial to study the parameters affecting the compounds and which doesn't, aiding in development with similar alterations done in the drugs. The chemists are groping in dark, whether which elements at certain positions may exhibit the electronic, steric and bonding effect. Inspite the drug is designed rationally yet luck plays an important role.

In some cases the series modifications in logical manner to the structure fails to enhance the activity significantly. Synthesizing such compounds in bulk and trying it with different modifications in structure may hit the luck. An evident of the luck synthesizing has been seen in sorafenib; an anticancer drug. This compound was found to be a bad in terms of activity when one substituent were present from possible two substituents, but the activity was improved when both were present and exhibited beneficial synergistic activity.

REFERENCES

L.P. Graham., An introduction to medicinal chemistry, 1st edition

K.R. Acharya., et al. ACE Revisited: A new target for structure-based drug design. Nature Reviews Drug Discovery (2003)

V.J. Hruby. Designing peptide receptor agonists and antagonists, Nature Reviews Drug Discovery, 847-858 (2002)

G.A. Jeffrey. Hydrogen bonding in biological structures, Springer-Verlag (1991)

J.T. Bolin., et al. Crystal structures of Escherichia coli and Lactobacillus casei dihydrofolate reductase refined at 1.7 A0 resolutions (1982)

A.R. Khan., et al. lowering the entropic barrier for binding conformationally flexible inhibitors to enzymes. Biochemistry, 16839-16845 (1998)

General features and binding of methotrexate (methotrexate binding). Journal of Biological Chemistry, 13650-13662

D.C. Rees., et al. Fragment based lead discovery, 660-672

S. Luca., et al. The conformation of neurotensin bound to its G protein-coupled receptor (active conformation by NMR), Proceedings of the National Academy of Sciences of the USA, 10706-10711 (2003)

M. Pellecchia., et al. NMR in drug discovery, Nature Reviews Drug Discovery, 211-219

E.G. Meyer., et al. Backward binding and other structural surprises. Perspectives in Drug discovery and Design, 168-195 (2002)

ABOUT THE AUTHOR

She is pursuing her studies in pharmacy and is keenly interested in medicinal chemistry. She hopes to satisfy the readers with her work. She believes that the only way to do great work is to love what you do.

"Poisons and medicines are often times the same substance given with different intents"- Humeera Rafeeq

www.ingramcontent.com/pod-product-compliance
Lightning Source LLC
Chambersburg PA
CBHW080522190526
45169CB00008B/3026
9781535419031